I0038696

HUMAN LEUKOCYTE ANTIGEN (HLA)

Edited by **Batool Mutar Mahdi**

Human Leukocyte Antigen (HLA)

http://dx.doi.org/10.5772/intechopen.73938

Edited by Batool Mutar Mahdi

Contributors

Shuyun Zhang, Tsukasa Nakamura, Takayuki Shirouzu, Norio Yoshimura, Hidetaka Ushigome, Maria Anagnostouli, Batool Mutar Mahdi

Notice

Statements and opinions expressed in the chapters are these of the individual contributors and not necessarily those of the editors or publisher. No responsibility is accepted for the accuracy of information contained in the published chapters. The publisher assumes no responsibility for any damage or injury to persons or property arising out of the use of any materials, instructions, methods or ideas contained in the book.

First published in London, United Kingdom, 2019 by IntechOpen

IntechOpen is the global imprint of INTECHOPEN LIMITED, registered in England and Wales, registration number: 11086078, The Shard, 25th floor, 32 London Bridge Street
London, SE19SG – United Kingdom
Printed in Croatia

British Library Cataloguing-in-Publication Data
A catalogue record for this book is available from the British Library

Additional hard copies can be obtained from orders@intechopen.com

Human Leukocyte Antigen (HLA), Edited by Batool Mutar Mahdi
p. cm.
Print ISBN 978-1-78985-761-0
Online ISBN 978-1-78985-762-7

We are IntechOpen,
the world's leading publisher of
Open Access books
Built by scientists, for scientists

4,000+
Open access books available

116,000+
International authors and editors

120M+
Downloads

151
Countries delivered to

Our authors are among the

Top 1%
most cited scientists

12.2%
Contributors from top 500 universities

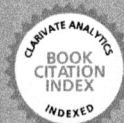

CLARIVATE ANALYTICS
BOOK CITATION INDEX
INDEXED

WEB OF SCIENCE™

Selection of our books indexed in the Book Citation Index
in Web of Science™ Core Collection (BKCI)

Interested in publishing with us?
Contact book.department@intechopen.com

Numbers displayed above are based on latest data collected.
For more information visit www.intechopen.com

Meet the editor

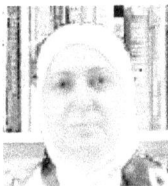

Professor Dr. Batool Mutar Mahdi is a medical doctor and consultant in clinical immunology. Previously she was head of the Human Leukocyte Antigen (HLA) tissue typing transplantation center in Al-Karamah Teaching Hospital-Ministry of Health and is now Head of the HLA Research Unit at Al-Kindy College of Medicine-Baghdad University. She currently works as a professor of clinical immunology at the same university. She has a Master's degree in Clinical Immunology and a board degree in Pathology-Clinical Immunology from the Iraqi Board of Clinical Specialization where she identified the HLA typing of the Iraqi population. She has published over 70 articles in peer-reviewed journals with a focus on the immunopathogenesis of many diseases. Most of her research deals with HLA and its association with diseases. Professor Dr. Batool is an international member of the American Society of Histocompatibility and Immunogenetics, European Society of Histocompatibility and Immunogenetics, and British Society of Immunology.

Contents

Preface

This book is a concise review of medically important applications of Human Leukocyte Antigen (HLA) in medicine. It covers both basic knowledge of HLA and its clinical applications in medical practice. Its two major aims are to assist students who are preparing for clinical immunology examinations, and to help people who want to understand more about this subject with brief and flexible sources of information. This book presents current, medically important information on the rapidly changing field of tissue typing and its relation with diseases. It includes updated information on such topics as tissue typing in medicine and transplantation. Our goal is to provide readers with an accurate source of clinically relevant information at different levels of medical education. These aims are achieved by utilizing different formats, which should make the book useful to students and readers with varying study objectives and learning styles. The information is presented succinctly with a stress on making it clear, interesting, and up to date.

We believe that readers appreciate a book that presents essential information in a readable and interesting format. We hope you find this book meets those criteria.

Finally, I would like to thank for my beloved mother for her kindness, endless support, and loving spirit that endure and sustain me; the memory of my darling father, a smart man whom I still miss every day; my adored brothers, Dr. Adil and Dr. Ali Ghalib; my wonderful nephew, Sajad; and our students, past, present, and future.

Professor Dr. Batool Mutar Mahdi
(MBChB, MSc, FICMS. Path-Clinical Immunology)
Consultant Clinical Immunology
Head of HLA Research Unit
Department of Microbiology
Al-Kindy College of Medicine
University of Baghdad, Iraq

Chapter 1

Introductory Chapter: Concept of Human Leukocyte Antigen (HLA)

Batool Mutar Mahdi

Additional information is available at the end of the chapter

http://dx.doi.org/10.5772/intechopen.83727

1. Introduction

The human leukocyte antigen (HLA) system is a cluster of gene complex encoding the major histocompatibility complex (MHC) proteins known as antigens located on the cell membrane of leukocytes in humans from which its name was derived. The functions of these cell surface proteins are many like responsible for the regulation of the immune system whether humoral or cellular in humans. It is the most important area in the vertebrate genome regarding infection and autoimmunity, and is essential in adaptive and innate immunity. The HLA gene complex is located on a 3-Mbp stretch within short arm of chromosome number 6p21. HLA genes are codominantly expressed and highly polymorphic, those have many different alleles that modify the adaptive immune system that helps body to distinguish the body's own protein from foreign invaders protein like virus, bacteria, or any other pathogens [1, 2].

1.1. Classification

The antigens of the HLA complex can be classified into three classes: class 1, class 2, and class 3.

1-MHC class I: There are three major and three minor MHC class I genes in HLA.

Major MHC class I:

- HLA-A
- HLA-B
- HLA-C

Minor MHC class I:

IntechOpen

- HLA-E

- HLA-F

HLA-G β_2-microglobulin binds with major and minor gene subunits to produce a heterodimer.

2-MHC class II: There are three major and two minor MHC class II proteins encoded by the HLA.

Major MHC class II:

1. HLA-DP

- α-chain encoded by HLA-DPA1 locus

- β-chain encoded by HLA-DPB1 locus

2. HLA-DQ

- α-chain encoded by HLA-DQA1 locus

- β-chain encoded by HLA-DQB1 locus

3. HLA-DR

- α-chain encoded by HLA-DRA locus

- β-chains (only three possible per person),

They are encoded by HLA-DRB1, DRB3, DRB4, and DRB5 loci.

The genes of the class II combine to form heterodimeric (αβ) protein receptors that are typically expressed on the surface of antigen-presenting cells.

Minor MHC class II:

- DM

- DO

They are used in the internal processing of antigens, loading the antigenic peptides generated from pathogens onto the HLA molecules of antigen-presenting cell [3, 4].

A person's HLA complex is genetically inherited from their parents (50% from each parent), so you are more likely to have stronger matches with your siblings than with a random member of the population; however, each pair of siblings still only has a 25% chance of matching perfectly. The likelihood of having a perfect match with someone unrelated to you is approximately 1 in 100,000. Thus, the closer the match between two people like identical twins, the less likely the recipient's immune system will attack the donor's cells (**Figure 1**) [5].

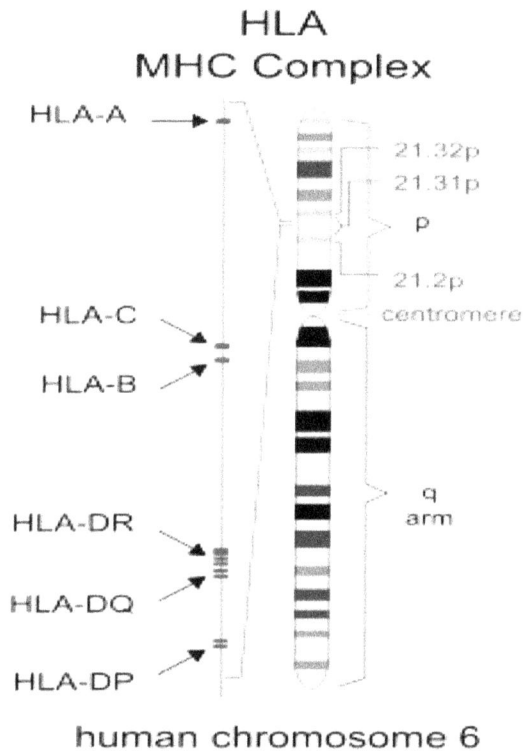

Figure 1. HLA complex is found on chromosome 6 in humans [5].

1.2. Structure

1.2.1. MHC class I

MHC class I molecule structure is consisting from two heterodimer polypeptide chains, α and β_2-microglobulin that linked together noncovalently by interaction of beta-2 microglobulin with α_3 domain of alpha chain. The alpha chain is encoded by many genes which are highly polymorphic, while beta-2 microglobulin subunit is not polymorphic and encoded by genes called beta-2 microglobulin gene. The other domain is α_3 domain which is plasma membrane that interacts with CD8 receptor of T-cytotoxic lymphocytes. This α_3-CD8 complex holds the MHC I molecule and the T-cell receptor (TCR) on the cell surface of the cytotoxic T cell binds its α_1-α_2 heterodimer and examines the foreign substance for antigenicity. The two domains, α_1 and α_2, fold to form a groove or basket for antigenic peptides to bind to it which consists of 8–10 amino acid in length (**Figure 2**) [6].

1.2.2. MHC class II

Class II molecules are also heterodimers in their structure, but consist of two homogenous peptides, an α and β polypeptide chain, both of which are encoded in the MHC. The alpha chain has two domes which are α_1 and α_2. Beta polypeptide chain has also two domains, β_1

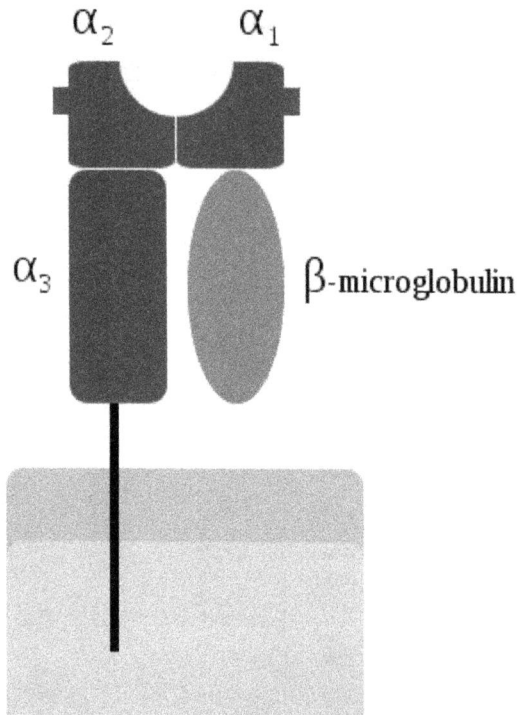

Figure 2. Structure of MHC class I.

and β_2. Every domain is encoded by a diverse exon gene, and other genes contain domains that encode different parts (leader sequences, transmembrane sequences, and cytoplasmic tail). The α_1 and β_1 regions of the chains form a membrane peptide binding domain, while the α_2 and β_2 regions form a membrane-proximal immunoglobulin-like domain. The groove or basket that binds the antigen or peptide is made up of two α-helix walls and β-sheet. Antigen-binding groove of MHC class II molecules is open at both ends and the groove on class I molecules is closed at each end resulting in antigens that bind to MHC class II molecules longer about 15–24 amino acid residues long. These domains are also highly polymorphic (**Figure 3**) [7].

1.3. Function

The major histocompatibility complex is a highly polymorphic region in the human genome located on short arm of chromosome number 6 about 200 genes in the region and is directly involved with the immune system. This is due to balancing selection acting on many genes with recombination in the MHC region [8]. These genes are in association with nonimmu-nologic genes like noncoding RNA genes, including expressed pseudogenes. MHC genes showed haplotype-specific linkage disequilibrium patterns contain the strongest cis- and trans-eQTLs/meQTLs in the genome and are called as a hot spot for disease associations.

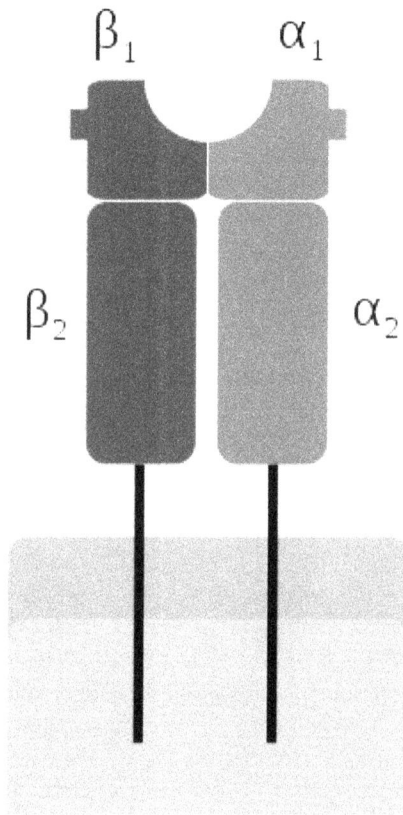

Figure 3. Structure of MHC class II.

The haplotype HLA-DR/DQ is structurally most variable and shows the highest number of disease associations. Dependence on a single reference sequence is not easy. Thus, analysis of GWAS for the MHC region is needed. One of the several issues with expected GWAS analysis is that it does not address this additional layer of polymorphisms unique to the MHC region [9]. Genome-wide association studies (GWAS) demonstrated that MHC is an important area for disease association, for example, autoimmune diseases [10, 11]. This very high-variety and broad-linkage disequilibrium leads to difficulty in assessing the one that leads to disease development and associations. Genome mapping can be sequence in addition to MHC haplotype and genome reference [12–14]. Many methods are defined but they are expensive [15–18]. Thus, many alleles of HLA had an association with cancer, infection with microorganisms in addition to its relation with transplant rejection.

1.4. Role of human leukocyte antigens (HLA) in transplantation

Human leukocyte antigens have an important role in graft rejection. One of the important squeal of mismatched graft is the development of donor-specific antibodies (DSA), which causes antibody-mediated rejection, graft loss, and repeat transplantation in addition to tissue typing. These DSA are induced by foreign epitopes present on the leukocytes mismatched with HLA antigens of the donor [19]. The presence of pretransplant DSAs in deceased donor transplantations is a risk marker for graft loss, whereas nondonor-specific anti-HLA antibodies are not associated with a lower graft survival and sensitized patients with these antibodies directed against class I and II may be a risk marker for graft loss in the long term [20]. These antibodies develop through pregnancy, blood transfusions, or organ transplants. After viral infection or vaccination, antibodies produced may have the capacity to cross-react with HLA called heterologous immunity caused by T-cell alloreactivity or by bystander activation of dormant HLA-specific memory B cells [21].

1.5. Human leukocyte antigen and disease association

HLA had an important role in immunopathogenesis of many diseases. The strongest association is HLA-B27 and ankylosing spondylitis. There is a long list of diseases associated with HLA. Bullous pemphigoid is the most common autoimmune blistering disease and is due to IgG recognition of two hemidesmosomal antigens, that is, BP230 (BP antigen 1) and BP180 (BP antigen 2, collagen XVII). The role of HLA-DQB1*03:01 binding to the immunogenic portion of BP180 provides a potential mechanism by which exposure to neuronal collagen BP180 may lead to cutaneous disease. Patients who have allele HLA-DQB1*03:01 had an increased T-cell avidity to many epitopes like BP180-NC16a domain. Patients with Th1/Th2 imbalance, anergy is absent and T-cells are subsequently primed end in autoimmunity against the BP180-NC16a domain and disease development [22]. Type 1 diabetes patients are more liable to develop celiac disease because these two diseases are associated with DQB1 *02:01 and DQB1 *03:02 and the patients with coexisting T1 diabetes and celiac disease had an HLA profile more similar to T1D patients than CeD patients [23].

Author details

Batool Mutar Mahdi

Address all correspondence to: abas_susan@yahoo.com

Department of Microbiology, Al-Kindy Medical College, University of Baghdad, Baghdad, Iraq

References

[1] Trowsdale J. Genomic structure and function in the MHC. Trends in Genetics. 1993; 9:117-122

[2] Horton R, Wilming L, Rand V, et al. Gene map of the extended human MHC. Nature Reviews. Genetics. 2004;5:889

[3] Milner CM, Campbell RD. Genes, genes and more genes in the human major histocom-patibility complex. BioEssays. 1992;**14**:565-571

[4] Shiina T, Inoko H, Kulski JK. An update of the HLA genomic region, locus information and disease associations: 2004. Tissue Antigens. 2004;**64**:631

[5] Rhodes DA, Trowsdale J. Genetics and molecular genetics of the MHC. Reviews in Immunogenetics. 1999;**1**:21-31

[6] Toh H, Savoie CJ, Kamikawaji N, Muta S, Sasazuki T, Kuhara S. Changes at the floor of the peptide-binding groove induce a strong preference for proline at position 3 of the bound peptide: Molecular dynamics simulations of HLA-A*0217. Biopolymers. 2000;**54**:318-327

[7] Jones EY, Fugger L, Strominger JL, Siebold C. MHC class II proteins and disease: A structural perspective. Nature Reviews. Immunology. 2006;**6**:271-282

[8] DeGiorgio M, Lohmueller KE, Nielsen R. A model-based approach for identifying sig-natures of ancient balancing selection in genetic data. PLoS Genetics. 2014;**10**:e1004561

[9] Kennedy AE, Ozbek U, Dorak MT. What has GWAS done for HLA and disease associa-tions? International Journal of Immunogenetics. 2017;**44**:195-211

[10] Trowsdale J, Knight JC. Major histocompatibility complex genomics and human disease. Annual Review of Genomics and Human Genetics. 2013;**14**:301-323

[11] Zhou F, Cao H, Zuo X, Zhang T, Zhang X, Liu X, et al. Deep sequencing of the MHC region in the Chinese population contributes to studies of complex disease. Nature Genetics. 2016;**48**:740-746

[12] Horton R, Gibson R, Coggill P, Miretti M, Allcock RJ, Almeida J, et al. Variation analysis and gene annotation of eight MHC haplotypes: The MHC haplotype project. Immunogenetics. 2008;**60**:1-18

[13] Dilthey A, Cox C, Iqbal Z, Nelson MR, McVean G. Improved genome inference in the MHC using a population reference graph. Nature Genetics. 2015;**47**:682-688

[14] Dilthey AT, Gourraud PA, Mentzer AJ, Cereb N, Iqbal Z, McVean G. High-accuracy HLA type inference from whole-genome sequencing data using population reference graphs. PLoS Computational Biology. 2016;**12**:e1005151

[15] Chaisson MJ, Huddleston J, Dennis MY, Sudmant PH, Malig M, Hormozdiari F, et al. Resolving the complexity of the human genome using single-molecule sequencing. Nature. 2015;**517**:608-611

[16] English AC, Salerno WJ, Hampton OA, Gonzaga-Jauregui C, Ambreth S, Ritter DI, et al. Assessing structural variation in a personal genome—Towards a human reference dip-loid genome. BMC Genomics. 2015;**16**:286

[17] Selvaraj S, Schmitt AD, Dixon JR, Ren B. Complete haplotype phasing of the MHC and KIR loci with targeted Haplo Seq. BMC Genomics. 2015;**16**:900

[18] Maretty L, Jensen JM, Petersen B, Sibbesen JA, Liu S, Villesen P, et al. Sequencing and de novo assembly of 150 genomes from Denmark as a population reference. Nature. 2017;**548**(7665):87-91

[19] Kramer CSM, Roelen DL, Heidt S, Claas FHJ. Defining the immunogenicity and antigenicity of HLA epitopes is crucial for optimal epitope matching in clinical renal transplantation. HLA. 2017;**90**:5-16

[20] Michielsen LA, Wisse BW, Kamburova EG, et al. A paired kidney analysis on the impact of pre-transplant anti-HLA antibodies on graft survival. Nephrology, Dialysis, Transplantation. 25 Oct. 2018. DOI: 10.1093/ndt/gfy316. [Epub ahead of print]

[21] Heidt S, Feltkamp MC, Karahan GE, et al. No evidence for cross-reactivity of virus-specific antibodies with HLA alloantigens. Transplantation. 2018;**102**:1844-1849

[22] Amber KT, Zikry J, Hertl M. A multi-hit hypothesis of bullous pemphigoid and associated neurological disease: Is HLA-DQB1*03:01, a potential link between immune privileged antigen exposure and epitope spreading? HLA. 2017;**89**:127-134

[23] Viken MK, Flåm ST, Skrivarhaug T, Amundsen SS, et al. HLA class II alleles in Norwegian patients with coexisting type 1 diabetes and celiac disease. HLA. 2017;**89**:278-284

Chapter 2

HLA Allele Frequencies in Pediatric and Adolescent Multiple Sclerosis Patients

Maria Anagnostouli and Maria Gontika

Additional information is available at the end of the chapter

http://dx.doi.org/10.5772/intechopen.81645

Abstract

Early-onset (pediatric and adolescent) multiple sclerosis (MS) is a chronic autoimmune and neurodegenerative disorder of the central nervous system, which accounts for 3–5% of all MS cases. The major histocompatibility complex (MHC) with its polymorphisms has been the genetic locus with the most robust association with adult MS, since its first discovery in the 1970s. Nowadays, human leukocyte antigen (HLA) typing studies and genome-wide association studies (GWAS) have tried to provide insight into the genetics of early-onset MS and their role in disease diagnosis, prognosis, and therapeutic decision-making. Fundamental genetic similarities have emerged, supporting the assumption that MS shares similar genetic variants and biological processes in all age groups. In this chapter, we considered it useful to collect all the available data concerning the HLA distribution in early-onset MS, given the absence of a review paper with such an approach. We additionally aimed toward the summarization of the association of the HLA frequencies in early-onset MS and the main acquired demyelinating disorders that are considered in differential diagnosis of early-onset MS, like ADEM, NMO/NMOSD, and anti-MOG encephalopathy, for further understanding and current or future research in this promising field.

Keywords: multiple sclerosis, pediatric, early onset, human leukocyte antigens, immunogenetics, therapy, precision medicine

1. Introduction

Early-onset (pediatric and adolescent) multiple sclerosis (MS), which accounts approximately for 3–5% of all MS cases worldwide, has recently aroused the interest of the scientific community regarding its underlying pathogenetic mechanisms, both autoimmune demyelination and neurodegeneration of the central nervous system (CNS) [1–3]. Additionally, in this

IntechOpen

specific age, other acquired demyelinating diseases are in the MS differential diagnosis of everyday practice, like ADEM, anti-MOG encephalopathy, and optic neuritis [4]. Recently, anti-NMO, anti-MOG, and other autoantibodies have been established as strong biomarkers of the previously referred newly emerged clinical entities or a key element of classical demyelinating diseases, like MS, especially of early onset [5, 6].

Nevertheless, for four decades now, the HLA alleles have been globally recognized as the core genetic (risk or protective) component in adult MS. Since the early 1970s, the major histocompatibility complex (MHC) with its polymorphisms on chromosome 6p21.3 [7, 8] has been the genetic locus with the most robust association with MS. In specific, DRB1*1501 (split of DR2), along with DRB1*0301 and DRB1*1301, has been found to confer risk for MS, while HLA-A*0201 protection against MS [9]. Genome-wide association studies (GWAS) regarding early-onset MS are still ongoing, in contrast with large-scale cohorts of adult-onset MS patients. However, single nucleotide polymorphisms (SNPs) of more modest effect have been detected that influence the risk of both adult- and early-onset MS, equalizing the genetic burden of these age groups [10–12]. The HLA alleles that have been studied in early-onset MS concern mainly the class II DRB1* and DQB1* loci, although DPB1* alleles confer susceptibility in adult-onset MS as well [13]. Thus, HLA immunogenetics in early-onset MS apart from the lower number of worldwide studies needs an extension to the whole HLA class I and class II systems, given the increased role that was in MS risk and MS association with vitamin D, body mass index (BMI), hormones, estrogen receptor, gender, EDSS score, disease course, MRI findings, cognitive status, and most importantly neutralizing antibody formation and response to treatment [8, 14–18].

In this chapter, we present the available data concerning the HLA distribution in early-onset MS, in parallel with the other acquired demyelinating diseases, given the increased knowledge that has recently emerged in this promising field. We also aimed to include all this useful data in a workable table.

2. HLA allele distribution in early-onset MS worldwide

Regarding HLA alleles, DRB1*15 association with early-onset MS has been noted by a series of studies [12, 19–22]. In 2000, a study of 286 Norwegians MS patients demonstrated that the HLA-DR2, DQ6 haplotype is negatively correlated with age at diagnosis [23]. Since then, many studies came to show that DRB1*15-positive patients have a significantly earlier age at onset than DRB1*15-negative patients [18, 24–30]. Maslova et al. replicated this testimony in a pure pediatric Russian population in 2000 [31]. An Australian study of 978 patients in 2010 went further to prove that carrying DRBI*15 significantly decreases the age of MS onset by 3.2 years in homozygotes and 1.3 years in heterozygotes [32].

On the other hand, a series of studies pleads against these remarks and claims no correlation of DRB1*15 status and age of disease onset [33–39]. In a Korean population, close linkage of DRB3*02, DRB1*13, and DQB1*03 was also associated with the risk of childhood MS, while DRB1*1501 was not as high as in Western children [40].

	MS	NMO	ADEM
HLA alleles	HLA-DRB1*1501 (Caucasian)	HLA-DRB1*03 (adult Caucasian)	HLA-DRB1*01 and HLA-DRB1*017 (Russian)
	HLA-DRB1*0401 (Caucasian)	HLA-DRB1*0501 (adult Japanese)	HLA-DRB1*1501 and HLA-DRB5*0101 (Korean)
	HLA-DRB3*02, HLA-DRB1*13, and HLA-DQB1*03 (Korean)		HLA-DQB1*0602, HLA-DRB1*1501, and HLA-DRB1*1503 (Brazil)
			HLA-DRB1*16 and HLA-DQB1*05 (Caucasian adult)

MS, multiple sclerosis; ADEM, acute disseminated encephalomyelitis; NMO, neuromyelitis optica.

Table 1. Summary of the available data regarding the HLA allele distribution in early-onset multiple sclerosis, ADEM, and NMO [12, 18–41, 46–49].

A remarkable DRB1-genotyping study in Australia in 2010 declared the first results indicative of the significance of the epistatic interactions at the HLA-DRB1 locus. Carriage of the DRB1*1501 risk allele alone was not significantly associated with age at disease onset, while the DRB1*0401 allele was associated with a reduced age at onset when combined with DRB1*1501 [41].

Regarding Greece, Anagnostouli et al. in 2003 noticed for the first time the higher frequency of DRB1*1501 in MS patients [42]. In 2011, Kouri et al. [43] observed no significant correlations among DRB1*1501, DQB1*0602, and DQA1*0102 alleles with age at onset, an observation repeated by Anagnostouli et al. in 2014 [20]. Anagnostouli et al. attributed this discrepancy either to a possible parent of origin effect, relying on Ramagopalan et al.' observation that only maternally transmitted DRB1*15 promotes a lower age of MS [44], or to fluctuations of vitamin D levels among different populations [45]. New findings in this former are the putative predisposing role of DRB1*03 allele and the protective role of the DRB1*16 allele for early-onset MS [20].

While the role of HLA alleles in early-onset MS has been well studied, this is not the case in other young-onset acquired demyelinating diseases, especially acute disseminated encephalomyelitis (ADEM) and neuromyelitis optica (NMO), its main differential diagnoses. In **Table 1**, we summarize the available data regarding the HLA allele distribution in early-onset MS, ADEM, and NMO, and despite the obvious lack of information, the primary results demonstrate clear genetic diversity [12, 18–41, 46–49].

3. Conclusions

The well-established HLA-DRB1*15:01 allele associated with adult-onset MS appears to confer increased susceptibility to early-onset MS too, supporting a fundamental similarity in genetic contribution to MS risk, regardless of age at onset. Regarding whether HLA-DRB1*1501 by itself lowers the age at onset of MS, the results are conflicting and possibly related to both genetic and environmental epistatic mechanisms and in particular those through HLA-DRB1*04. Moreover,

HLA-DRB1*04 also appears to bind with high affinity to myelin oligodendrocyte glycoprotein (MOG) epitopes, whose role in early-onset demyelinating disorders has been widely studied, in both familial MS patients and asymptomatic relatives, indicating that the humoral immune reactivity against MOG is partially under control of certain HLA class II alleles [50–54]. This observation could guide therapy, as HLA-DRB1∗0401 allele is associated with greater risk of developing neutralizing antibodies against interferon beta (IFN-β) in adult studies, resulting in poorer therapeutic outcome [55]. Finally, the putative relation of DRB1*03 allele with early-onset MS is also interesting, as this allele has been associated not only with a presumed better MS prognosis but also with NMO [46], a mainly humoral immunological entity.

Accumulating data highlights the role of HLA-genotype and especially HLA-DRB1*1501 in regulating the immune response to a range of environmental factors, modulating the risk of MS appearance. Research has mainly focused on viral infections, especially EBV [56–58], CMV, and HSV-1 [58]. In specific, Epstein–Barr nuclear antigen-1 seropositivity has been associated with an increased risk of MS, while a remote infection with CMV with a lower risk. A strong interaction has been found between HSV-1 status and HLA-DRB1 in predicting MS, as HSV-1 has been associated with an increased risk of MS only in DRB1*15 carriers. Moreover, obesity and higher body mass index (BMI) during adolescence, rather than childhood, seem to be critical in determining MS risk [59], while tobacco smoke exposure and HLA-DRB1*15 interact to increase risk for MS in children diagnosed with monophasic acquired demyelinating syndromes [60]. Finally, as research regarding the role of gut bacteria in the development of central nervous demyelinating disorders robustly expands, possible protective correlations of specific bacteria through interplay with specific HLA alleles emerge in animal models of MS, expanding our knowledge regarding disease pathogenesis [61, 62]. Larger studies in early-onset MS populations are required in order to clarify these possible correlations which may also expand to other HLA alleles, proving the interplay among cellular activity, humoral activity, and environment in MS and their possible impact in therapeutics.

In conclusion, HLA alleles emerge as a primary biomarker in both early- and adult-onset MS, regarding genetic risk, outcome, and differential diagnosis. We strongly believe that larger HLA-genotyping studies regarding early-onset demyelinating disorders are needed, in different ethnic groups, in order to clarify, replicate, and expand the already limited existing results. We also believe that these future studies will aim toward personalized therapeutics and generally precision medicine in early-onset MS patients.

Author details

Maria Anagnostouli[1,2]* and Maria Gontika[1]

*Address all correspondence to: managnost@med.uoa.gr

1 Immunogenetics Laboratory, 1st Dep. of Neurology, Medical School, National and Kapodistrian University of Athens, Athens, Greece

2 Demyelinating Diseases Clinic, 1st Dep. of Neurology, Medical School, National and Kapodistrian University of Athens, Athens, Greece

References

[1]   Renoux C, Vukusic S, Confavreux C. The natural history of multiple sclerosis with child-hood onset. Clinical Neurology and Neurosurgery. 2008;**110**(9):897-904

[2]   Venkateswaran S, Banwell B. Pediatric multiple sclerosis. The Neurologist. 2010;**16**(2): 92-105

[3]   Ferreira ML, Machado MI, Dantas MJ, Moreira AJ, Souza AM. Pediatric multiple sclerosis: Analysis of clinical and epidemiological aspects according to National MS Society consensus 2007. Arquivos de Neuro-Psiquiatria. 2008;**66**(3B):665-670

[4]   Hintzen RQ, Dale RC, Neuteboom RF, et al. Pediatric acquired CNS demyelinating syndromes: Features associated with multiple sclerosis. Neurology. 2016;**87**(9 Suppl 2): S67-S73

[5]   Chitnis T, Ness J, Krupp L, et al. Clinical features of neuromyelitis optica in children: US network of pediatric MS centers report. Neurology. 2016;**86**(3):245-252

[6]   Hennes EM, Baumann M, Lechner C, et al. MOG Spectrum disorders and role of MOG-antibodies in clinical practice. Neuropediatrics. 2018;**49**(1):3-11

[7]   Ramagopalan SV, Dyment DA, Ebers GC. Genetic epidemiology: The use of old and new tools for multiple sclerosis. Trends in Neurosciences. 2008;**31**:645-652

[8]   Katsavos S, Anagnostouli M. Biomarkers in multiple sclerosis: An up-to-date overview. Multiple Sclerosis International. 2013;**2013**:340508

[9]   International Multiple Sclerosis Genetics Consortium; Welcome Trust Case Control Consortium 2, Sawcer S, Hellenthal G, Pirinen M, Spencer CC, et al. Genetic risk and a primary role for cell-mediated immune mechanisms in multiple sclerosis. Nature. 2011;**476**:214-219

[10] Disanto G, Ramagopalan SV. Similar genetics of adult and pediatric MS: Age is just a number. Neurology. 2013;**81**(23):1974-1975

[11] Graves JS, Barcellos LF, Simpson S, et al. The multiple sclerosis risk allele within the AHI1 gene is associated with relapses in children and adults. Multiple Sclerosis Related Disorders. 2018;**19**:161-165

[12] Gianfrancesco MA, Stridh P, Shao X, et al. Genetic risk factors for pediatric-onset multiple sclerosis. Multiple Sclerosis. 2017;**1**:1352458517733551

[13] Patsopoulos NA, Barcellos LF, Hintzen RQ, et al. Fine-mapping the genetic association of the major histocompatibility complex in multiple sclerosis: HLA and non-HLA effects. PLoS Genetics. 2013;**9**(11):e1003926

[14] Sintzel MB, Rametta M, Reder AT, et al. Vitamin D and multiple sclerosis: A comprehensive review. Neurology and Therapy. 2018;**7**(1):59-85

[15] Hedström AK, Lima Bomfim I, Barcellos L, et al. Interaction between adolescent obesity and HLA risk genes in the etiology of multiple sclerosis. Neurology. 2014;**82**(10):865-872

[16] Kikuchi S, Fukazawa T, Niino M, et al. Estrogen receptor gene polymorphism and multiple sclerosis in Japanese patients: Interaction with HLA-DRB1*1501 and disease modulation. Journal of Neuroimmunology. 2002;**128**(1-2):77-81

[17] Katsavos S, Artemiadis A, Davaki P, et al. Familial multiple sclerosis in Greece: Distinct clinical and imaging characteristics in comparison with the sporadic disease. Clinical Neurology and Neurosurgery. 2018;**173**:144-149

[18] Okuda DT, Srinivasan R, Oksenberg JR, et al. Genotype-phenotype correlations in multiple sclerosis: HLA genes influence disease severity inferred by 1HMR spectroscopy and MRI measures. Brain. 2009;**132**(Pt 1):250-259

[19] Stamatelos P, Anagnostouli M. HLA-genotype in multiple sclerosis: The role in disease onset, clinical course, cognitive status and response to treatment: A clear step towards personalized therapeutics. Immunogenetics Open Access. 2017;**2**:116. (review in press)

[20] Anagnostouli M, Manouseli A, Artemiadis A, et al. HLA-DRB1* allele frequencies in pediatric, adolescent and adult-onset multiple sclerosis patients, in a Hellenic sample. Evidence for new and established associations. Multiple Sclerosis Journal. 2014;**1**:1

[21] Banwell B, Bar-Or A, Arnold DL, et al. Clinical, environmental, and genetic determinants of multiple sclerosis in children with acute demyelination: A prospective national cohort study. Lancet Neurology. 2011;**10**(5):436-445

[22] Disanto G, Magalhaes S, Handel AE, et al. HLA-DRB1 confers increased risk of pediatric-onset MS in children with acquired demyelination. Neurology. 2011;**76**(9):781-786

[23] Celius EG, Harbo HF, Egeland T, et al. Sex and age at diagnosis are correlated with the HLA-DR2, DQ6 haplotype in multiple sclerosis. Journal of the Neurological Sciences. 2000;**178**(2):132-135

[24] Masterman T, Ligers A, Olsson T, et al. HLA-DR15 is associated with lower age at onset in multiple sclerosis. Annals of Neurology. 2000;**48**(2):211-219

[25] Hensiek AE, Sawcer SJ, Feakes R, et al. HLA-DR 15 is associated with female sex and younger age at diagnosis in multiple sclerosis. Journal of Neurology, Neurosurgery, and Psychiatry. 2002;**72**(2):184-187

[26] Weatherby SJ, Thomson W, Pepper L, et al. HLA-DRB1 and disease outcome in multiple sclerosis. Journal of Neurology. 2001;**248**(4):304-310

[27] Smestad C, Brynedal B, Jonasdottir G, et al. The impact of HLA-A and -DRB1 on age at onset, disease course and severity in Scandinavian multiple sclerosis patients. European Journal of Neurology. 2007;**14**(8):835-840

[28] Imrell K, Greiner E, Hillert J, Masterman T. HLA-DRB115 and cerebrospinal-fluid-specific oligoclonal immunoglobulin G bands lower age at attainment of important disease milestones in multiple sclerosis. Journal of Neuroimmunology. 2009;**210**(1-2):128-130

[29] Balnyte R, Rastenyte D, Vaitkus A, et al. The importance of HLA DRB1 gene allele to clinical features and disability in patients with multiple sclerosis in Lithuania. BMC Neurology. 2013;**13**:77

[30] Al-Shammri S, Nelson RF, Al-Muzairi I, Akanji AO. HLA determinants of susceptibility to multiple sclerosis in an Arabian gulf population. Multiple Sclerosis. 2004;**10**(4):381-386

[31] Maslova OI, Bykova OV, Guseva MR, et al. Multiple sclerosis with early onset: Pathogenesis, clinical characteristics, possibilities in the treatment of its pathogenesis. Zhurnal Nevrologii i Psikhiatrii Imeni S.S. Korsakova. 2002;(Suppl):46-51

[32] Van der Walt A, Stankovich J, Bahlo M, et al. Heterogeneity at the HLA-DRB1 allelic variation locus does not influence multiple sclerosis disease severity, brain atrophy or cognition. Multiple Sclerosis. 2011;**17**(3):344-352

[33] Villoslada P, Barcellos LF, Rio J, et al. The HLA locus and multiple sclerosis in Spain. Role in disease susceptibility, clinical course and response to interferon beta. Journal of Neuroimmunology. 2002;**130**(1-2):194-201

[34] Barcellos LF, Sawcer S, Ramsay PP, et al. Heterogeneity at the HLA-DRB1 locus and risk for multiple sclerosis. Human Molecular Genetics. 2006;**15**(18):2813-2824

[35] Barcellos LF, Oksenberg JR, Begovich AB, et al. HLA-DR2 dose effect on susceptibility to multiple sclerosis and influence on disease course. American Journal of Human Genetics. 2003;**72**(3):710-716

[36] Silva AM, Pereira C, Bettencourt A, et al. The role of HLA-DRB1 alleles on susceptibility and outcome of a Portuguese multiple sclerosis population. Journal of the Neurological Sciences. 2007;**258**(1-2):69-74

[37] Ouadghiri S, El Alaoui Toussi K, Brick C, et al. Genetic factors and multiple sclerosis in the Moroccan population: A role for HLA class II. Pathologie Biologie. 2013;**61**(6):259-263

[38] Ballerini C, Guerini FR, Rombolà G, et al. HLA-multiple sclerosis association in continental Italy and correlation with disease prevalence in Europe. Journal of Neuroimmunology. 2004;**150**(1-2):178-185

[39] Boiko AN, Gusev EI, Sudomoina MA, et al. Association and linkage of juvenile MS with HLA-DR2(15) in Russians. Neurology. 2002;**58**(4):658-660

[40] Oh HH, Kwon SH, Kim CW, et al. Molecular analysis of HLA class II-associated susceptibility to neuroinflammatory diseases in Korean children. Journal of Korean Medical Science. 2004;**19**:426-430

[41] Wu JS, Qiu W, Castley A, et al. Modifying effects of HLA-DRB1 allele interactions on age at onset of multiple sclerosis in Western Australia. Multiple Sclerosis. 2010;**16**(1):15-20

[42] Bozikas VP, Anagnostouli MC, Petrikis P, et al. Familial bipolar disorder and multiple sclerosis: A three-generation HLA family study. Progress in Neuro-Psychopharmacology & Biological Psychiatry. 2003;**27**(5):835-839

[43] Kouri I, Papakonstantinou S, Bempes V, et al. HLA associations with multiple sclerosis in Greece. Journal of the Neurological Sciences. 2011;**308**(1-2):28-31

[44] Ramagopalan SV, Byrnes JK, Dyment DA, et al. Parent-of-origin of HLA-DRB1*1501 and age of onset of multiple sclerosis. Journal of Human Genetics. 2009;**54**(9):547-549

[45] Ramagopalan SV, Maugeri NJ, Handunnetthi L, et al. Expression of the multiple scle-rosis-associated MHC class II allele HLA-DRB1*1501 is regulated by vitamin D. PLoS Genetics. 2009;**5**:e1000369

[46] Gontika M, Anagnostouli M. Human leukocyte antigens immunogenetics of neuromye-litis optica or Devic's disease and the impact on the immunopathogenesis, diagnosis and treatment: A critical review. Neuroimmunology and Neuroinflammation. 2014;**1**:44-50

[47] Imbesi D, Calabrò RS, Gervasi G, et al. Does HLA class II haplotype play a role in adult acute disseminated encephalomyelitis? Preliminary findings from a southern Italy hospital-based study. Archives Italiennes de Biologie. 2012;**150**(1):1-4

[48] Alves-Leon SV, Veluttini-Pimentel ML, Gouveia ME, et al. Acute disseminated encepha-lomyelitis: Clinical features, HLA DRB1*1501, HLA DRB1*1503, HLA DQA1*0102, HLA DQB1*0602, and HLA DPA1*0301 allelic association study. Arquivos de Neuro-Psiquiatria. 2009;**67**(3A):643-651

[49] Idrissova ZR, Boldyreva MN, Dekonenko EP, et al. Acute disseminated encephalomyeli-tis in children: Clinical features and HLA-DR linkage. European Journal of Neurology. 2003;**10**(5):537-546

[50] Forsthuber TG, Shive CL, Wienhold W, et al. T cell epitopes of human myelin oligodendro-cyte glycoprotein identified in HLA-DR4 (DRB1*0401) transgenic mice are encephalito-genic and are presented by human B cells. Journal of Immunology. 2001;**167**(12):7119-7125

[51] Klehmet J, Shive C, Guardia-Wolff R, et al. T cell epitope spreading to myelin oligoden-drocyte glycoprotein in HLA-DR4 transgenic mice during experimental autoimmune encephalomyelitis. Clinical Immunology. 2004;**111**(1):53-60

[52] Khare M, Rodriguez M, David CS. HLA class II transgenic mice authenticate restriction of myelin oligodendrocyte glycoprotein-specific immune response implicated in mul-tiple sclerosis pathogenesis. International Immunology. 2003;**15**(4):535-546

[53] Raddassi K, Kent SC, Yang J, et al. Increased frequencies of myelin oligodendrocyte gly-coprotein/MHC class II-binding CD4 cells in patients with multiple sclerosis. Journal of Immunology. 2011;**187**(2):1039-1046

[54] Lutterotti A, Reindl M, Gassner C, et al. Antibody response to myelin oligodendrocyte glycoprotein and myelin basic protein depend on familial background and are partially associated with human leukocyte antigen alleles in multiplex families and sporadic mul-tiple sclerosis. Journal of Neuroimmunology. 2002;**131**(1-2):201-207

[55] Buck D, Cepok S, Hoffmann S, et al. Influence of the HLADRB1 genotype on antibody development to interferon beta in multiple sclerosis. Archives of Neurology. 2011;**68**(4): 480-487

[56] Waubant E, Mowry EM, Krupp L, et al. Antibody response to common viruses and human leukocyte antigen-DRB1 in pediatric multiple sclerosis. Multiple Sclerosis. 2013;**19**(7): 891-895

[57] Morandi E, Jagessar SA, 't Hart BA, Gran B. EBV infection empowers human B cells for autoimmunity: Role of autophagy and relevance to multiple sclerosis. Journal of Immunology. 2017;**199**(2):435-448

[58] Waubant E, Mowry EM, Krupp L, et al. Common viruses associated with lower pediatric multiple sclerosis risk. Neurology. 2011;**76**(23):1989-1995

[59] Hedström AK, Olsson T, Alfredsson L. Body mass index during adolescence, rather than childhood, is critical in determining MS risk. Multiple Sclerosis. 2016;**22**(7):878-883

[60] Lavery AM, Collins BN, Waldman AT, et al. The contribution of secondhand tobacco smoke exposure to pediatric multiple sclerosis risk. Multiple Sclerosis. 2018;**1**:1352458518757089

[61] Mangalam A, Shahi SK, Luckey D, et al. Human gut-derived commensal bacteria suppress CNS inflammatory and demyelinating disease. Cell Reports. 2017;**20**(6):1269-1277

[62] Lerner A, Matthias T. Rheumatoid arthritis-celiac disease relationship: Joints get that gut feeling. Autoimmunity Reviews. 2015;**14**(11):1038-1047

Donor-Specific Anti-HLA Antibodies in Organ Transplantation: Transition from Serum DSA to Intra-Graft DSA

Tsukasa Nakamura, Hidetaka Ushigome,
Takayuki Shirouzu and Norio Yoshimura

Additional information is available at the end of the chapter

http://dx.doi.org/10.5772/intechopen.79846

Abstract

In the field of organ transplantation, donor-specific anti-HLA antibodies (DSA) have gained more popularity, as antibody-mediated rejection (AMR) has been recognized as an important factor to determine allograft survival. Thus, it is reasonable to believe that appropriate control of DSA is directly linked to well-managed immunosuppression, resulting in free from AMR. First, in order to prevent and manage AMR, it is of vital importance to be familiar with updated knowledge regarding crossmatch test and DSA detection methods, including intra-graft DSA. Second, it is also crucial to understand the standard criteria to diagnose AMR. Although pathological diagnosis and serum DSA (s-DSA) detection play the central role, the recent trend seems to be detection of intra-graft DSA (g-DSA). Third, regarding organ transplantation between sensitized pairs, the acceptable outcomes are obtained owing to recent preoperative desensitization protocols: depletion/modification of B cells, apheresis for antibodies, and inhibition of reaction between DSA and HLA. Finally, we would like to discuss the treatment of AMR. Further advances in diagnosis methods and emergences of effective treatments would be expected for acceptable control of AMR. In this chapter, we will review from the basics to recent topics in order to understand DSA and AMR.

Keywords: organ transplantation, antibody-mediated rejection, donor-specific anti-HLA antibodies, intra-graft donor-specific anti-HLA antibodies, immunocomplex capture fluorescence analysis

1. Introduction

Recent advances in immunosuppression permit for organ transplantation between sensitized recipients and donors with acceptable outcomes. However, it is true that the management of acute or, in particular, chronic antibody-mediated rejection (AMR) due to donor-specific anti-HLA antibodies (DSA) is still a crucial issue to improve long-term graft survival. Because chronic changes of AMR are irreversible, it is also true that an early accurate diagnosis of AMR is required to prevent severe consequences. Thus, it is reasonable to believe that DSA is a main research topic to improve the outcome of organ transplantation. In the 1960s, the introduction of azathioprine brought the beginning of contemporary organ transplantation [1]. Following this era, incompatibilities, anti-AB [2, 3] and anti-HLA antibodies [4], were recognized as a crucial barrier for organ transplantation. In the next half-century, the main attention was paid to cellular rejection: T-cell-mediated rejection [5]. This resulted in the development of calcineurin inhibitors [6] and several antibody drugs [7]: a depletion of lymphocytes that enabled the control of T-cell-mediated rejection. However, AMR remains an important issue that is still not addressed. Then, DSA have finally received strong attention in the twenty-first century because DSA are important factors to determine long-term graft survival. In this chapter, we will review DSA in organ transplantation and discuss effectiveness of a novel application of immunocomplex capture fluorescence analysis (ICFA), as well as crossmatch examinations, protocols of desensitization, and outcomes of crossmatch positive organ transplantation.

2. Assessment for donor-specific anti-HLA antibodies

To assess reactive DSA in recipient serum, a crossmatch test or measurement of DSA is performed routinely in clinical organ transplantation. There are several crossmatch methods: lymphocyte cytotoxic test (LCT), flow cytometry crossmatch (FCXM), and ICFA. In addition to crossmatch test, antibody detection methods such as flow PRA screening and single antigen bead assay (SAB) are utilized in clinical settings. Generally, it is important to understand the advantages and disadvantages of these methods and interpret appropriately.

2.1. Lymphocyte cytotoxic test

Antigen–antibody and complement-dependent reactions are observed in this traditional direct-crossmatch test. Donor lymphocytes are incubated in the recipient serum, followed by the addition of complements. Under the circumstances where there are DSA in the recipient serum, lymphocytes are necrotized by the complement-dependent cytotoxicity reaction. Then, adding eosin dye, the ratio of necrotized lymphocytes is counted by a phase-contrast microscopy (**Figure 1**). The disadvantages of LCT are relatively low sensitivity, difficulty in obtaining donor alive lymphocytes, and subjective judges. Furthermore, it should be noted that sometimes non-DSA reaction can be observed. Conversely, only this traditional method is capable of visualizing real reactions against donor cells, including non-DSA reactions [8]. Thus, it is true that careful attention should be paid when positive reaction in LCT is detected [9].

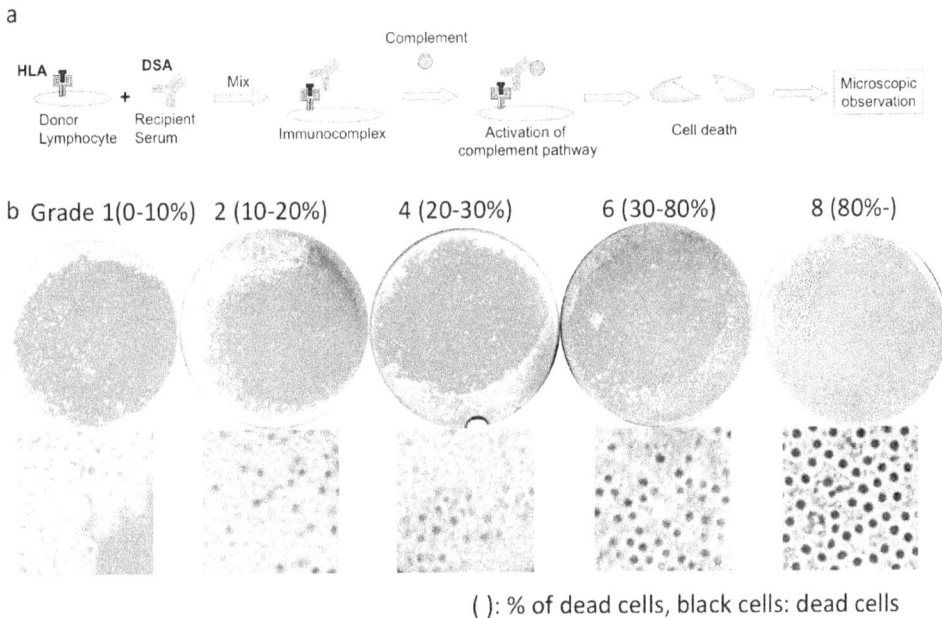

Figure 1. Lymphocyte cytotoxicity test (LCT). (a) Schematic presentation of LCT. (b) Representative results of LCT. Necrotized lymphocytes were stained in black by eosin dye. Negative reaction (grade 1–2) and positive reaction (grade 4–8).

2.2. Flow cytometry crossmatch

FCXM is an examination that flow cytometry technology is applied. As characteristics of FCXM test, sensitivity is high enough to detect a slight amount of DSA. Therefore, it should be paid attention that non-HLA antibodies might be detected: false positive. Because of high-sensitivity examination, rigorous quality control is required. To apply FCXM, donor lymphocytes and recipient serum samples were utilized. Subsequently, antihuman IgG antibodies are added and positivity is determined [10]. In addition, to add CD3 or CD19, T cells and B cells can be separated and analyzed simultaneously (**Figure 2**).

2.3. Immunocomplex capture fluorescence analysis

WAKFlow HLA antibody class I and II ICFA (Wakunaga Pharmaceutical Co., Ltd., Osaka, Japan) is one of the crossmatch tests by using donor lymphocytes and recipient serum [11]. This technique can detect DSA immunocomplex with high specificity [12]. As a detection system, Luminex xMAP technology (Luminex Corporation, Austin, TX) is applied. Schematic presentation of ICFA is shown in **Figure 3**. First, HLA and DSA complexes are formed following the reaction between donor lymphocytes and recipient serum containing DSA. Second, lymphocytes are lysed and complexes remain in lysates. Third, these complexes are captured by anti-HLA monoclonal antibodies fixed on Luminex beads, and subsequently PE-conjugated human anti-IgG is added. Finally, Luminex system detects these PE-conjugated anti-human

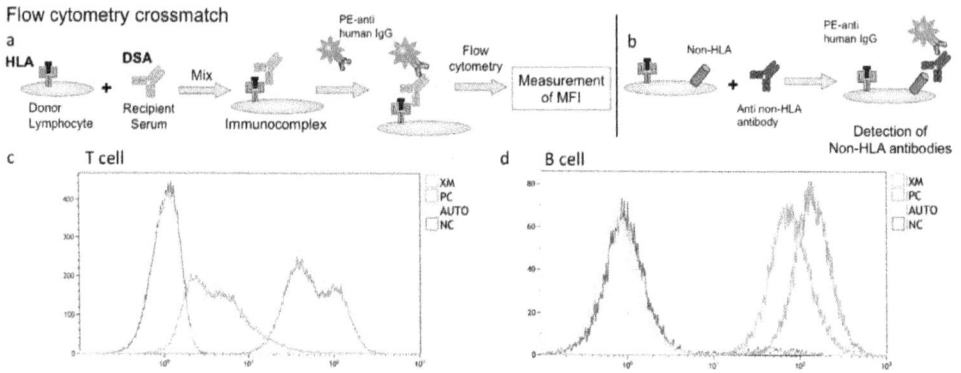

Figure 2. Flow cytometry crossmatch (FCXM). (a) Schematic presentation of FCXM. (b) an example of positive reaction by non-HLA antibodies. (c), (d) representative results of FCXM using T cell (c) or B cell (d).

Immunocomplex Capture Fluorescence Analysis

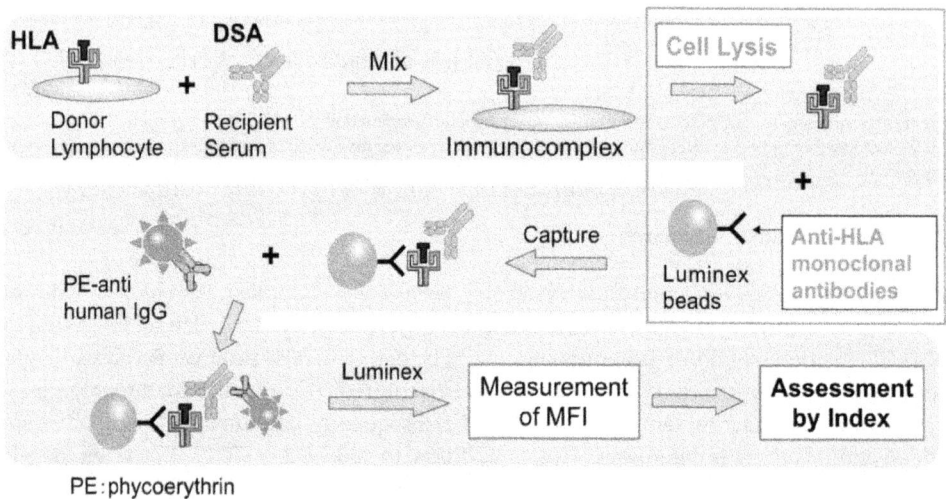

PE : phycoerythrin

Figure 3. Schematic presentation of immunocomplex capture fluorescence analysis (ICFA).

IgG signals. As ICFA characteristics, the following features are noted: (1) the specificity of identifying HLA antibodies is high, and (2) class I and II antibodies can be identified separately. Furthermore, in terms of recent advances in ICFA, DR, DQ, and DP, DSA can be identified separately.

2.4. FlowPRA screening

To identify anti-HLA antibodies in serum, FlowPRA screening test is performed. First, a reaction is caused between anti-HLA antibodies and latex beads coated with HLA antigens. Then,

FITC-conjugated antihuman IgG is added. Subsequently, mean fluorescence intensity (MFI) and shift from negative control are calculated based on flow cytometry analyses (**Figure 4**). Each mixed class I and II HLA antigen is separately coated on latex beads, derived from about 30 types of panel cells [13]. Depending on the human race, there is a possibility that rare HLA

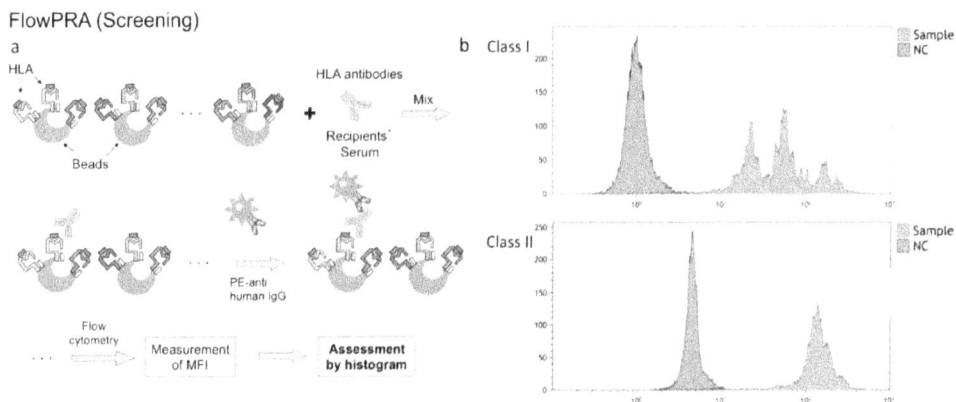

Figure 4. FlowPRA screening. (a) Schematic presentation of FlowPRA screening. (b) Examples of positive FlowPRA screening results about class I (upper) and class II (lower).

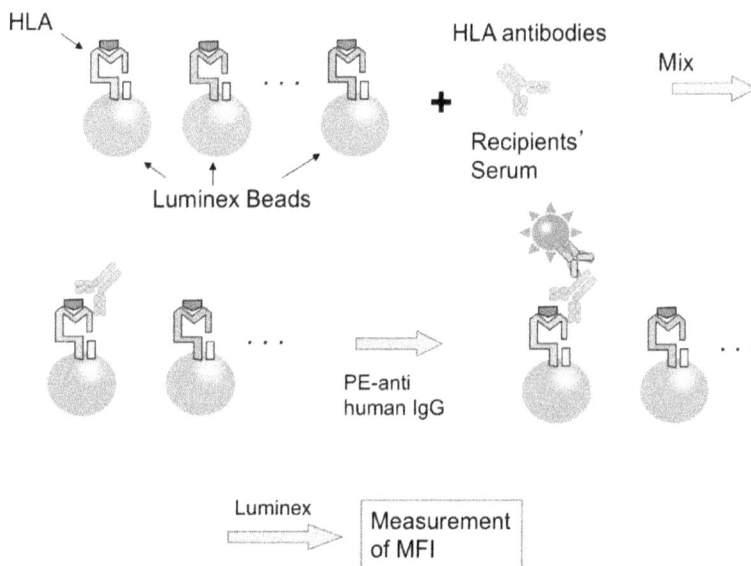

Figure 5. Schematic presentation of single antigen bead assay (SAB).

antigens are not covered. These disadvantages should be recognized. Generally, if a positive reaction would be observed, the following SAB is applied to identify the specificity of anti-HLA antibodies.

2.5. Single antigen bead assay

To identify the specificity of anti-HLA antibodies, SAB is performed when crossmatch test and/or FlowPRA is positive. First, a reaction is observed between anti-HLA antibodies and Luminex beads coated with a single HLA antigen extracted from gene-modified cells. Following steps are similar to those of FCXM. Finally, these reactions, MFI of PE signals, were calculated by Luminex system (Luminex Corporation). According to HLA typing of donor, the presence of DSA is judged. It is often used in LABScreen single antigen HLA class I/II beads: LABScreen single antigen class I/LABScreen single antigen class II (One Lambda Inc., Canoga Park, CA) or WAKFlow HLA antibody class I HR and WAKFlow HLA antibody class II HR (Wakunaga Pharmaceutical Co., Ltd) (**Figure 5**). As an important point, because these single HLA antigen beads do not include all types of HLA antigens, we should be familiar with SAB kit to judge the existence of DSA appropriately.

3. Assessment for intra-graft donor-specific anti-HLA antibodies

Due to recent advances in examinations for DSA, the assessment for g-DSA has been paid attention. In fact, it is hard to understand that s-DSA damage allografts without localization in target organs. Thus, hereafter, the assessment of g-DSA would gain more popularity as diagnosis or prognosis factors. Although the presence of g-DSA is not included in AMR diagnosis criteria currently, g-DSA might be a key criterion for considering AMR in the near future. It would be better that clinicians and researchers are aware of this novel topic. Here, we will present representative two different methods. We will also delve into graft ICFA technique in this section.

3.1. Dissociation between HLA and DSA (acid elution method)

To obtain free DSA from allografts, dissociation HLA and DSA complexes are attempted. So far, g-DSA detection in the kidney [14–16], liver [17], and lung [18] were reported. This method requires the following steps: (1) Wash more than seven times to prevent from detection s-DSA incorrectly. (2) Dissociate these complexes by acid (buffer). (3) Detect dissociated DSA by SAB (**Figure 6**). As compared to graft ICFA, mentioned later, acid elution method has weak points regarding simplicity and remains doubtful points whether DSA denature or not during the acid elution step. However, SAB analysis following acid elution seems to be accepted widely and allows to identify specific DSA even where multiple candidate DSA exist. The common recognition of g-DSA assessment seems to be that g-DSA is an important factor to determine graft survival and more sensitive than s-DSA [14].

3.2. Graft immunocomplex capture fluorescence analysis (non-dissociation technique)

WAKFlow HLA antibody class I and II ICFA is an attractive tool to identify HLA/DSA complexes as mentioned above, by means of WAKFlow HLA antibody class I and II (Wakunaga

acid elution method

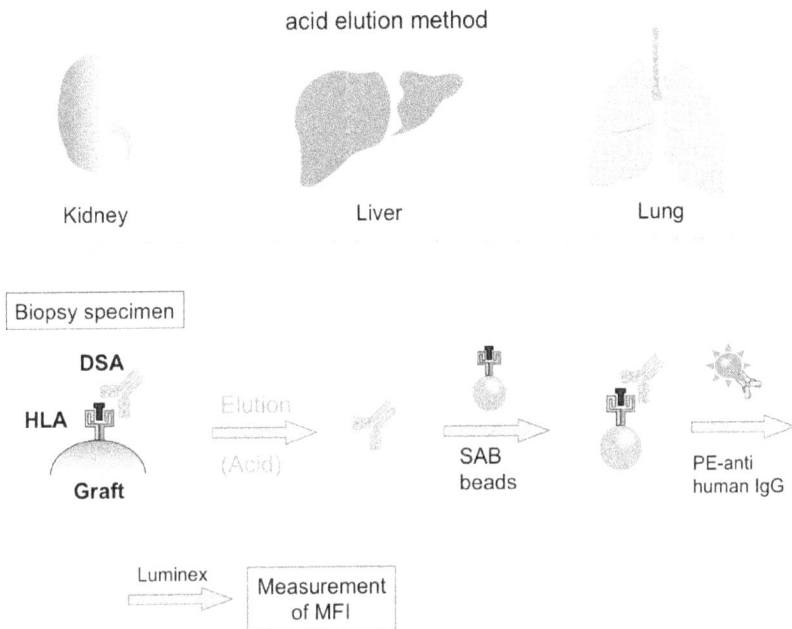

Figure 6. The flowchart of the acid elution method (dissociation technique).

Pharmaceutical). It is not only for serum of recipients but also for allograft specimens. The first graft ICFA was introduced as an effective tool for detection of g-DSA in 2017 [19, 20]. Graft ICFA can be performed as previously described by Nakamura et al. Graft samples were obtained by means of a percutaneous needle biopsy. To standardize the results of graft ICFA, 2 mm specimen was used for each analysis. Regarding graft ICFA to identify HLA expression, samples were washed enough in PBS. As compared to acid elution method of DSA from grafts associated to g-DSA detection by SAB, graft ICFA does not allow to identify individual responsible HLA alleles, such as HLA-A24, etc. However, in the setting of real organ transplantation, generally HLA alleles are identified prior to transplantation. Thus, it does not seem to be difficult to narrow down candidate HLA. It is true, therefore, that current graft ICFA is clinically useful to diagnose AMR. Moreover, the combination of acid elution method and graft ICFA allows to obtain useful information regarding g-DSA. Further advances in graft ICFA would be expected.

(Ethics Committee approval was obtained from the internal research ethics committee of Kyoto Prefectural University of Medicine. The clinical trial registration number is UMIN000023787.)

3.3. Data interpretation

MFI of samples was calculated by the Luminex system. A ratio of sample MFI/blank beads MFI of all negative samples, including HLA matched recipients' samples, + 2SD is demonstrated below 0.9 (data not shown) (please refer to [19, 20]). Then the ratio was determined, and ≥ 1.0 was considered as a positive result. Furthermore, to compensate baseline reaction, the following index was also calculated. Index = $(X_{HLA}-(N_{HLA}-N_{BB})X_{BB}/N_{BB})/X_{BB}$: X_{HLA}, sample

MFI; X_{BB}, sample blank beads MFI; N_{HLA}, the mean MFI of negative samples; and N_{BB}, the mean blank beads MFI of negative samples. Given the results of negative samples, the index ≥ 1.5 was considered as a positive result.

3.4. DSA-HLA complexes in the liver, heart, lungs, pancreas, and small intestine are also successfully detected by graft ICFA

To confirm whether graft ICFA can be applied to other organs besides the kidney [19, 20], we employed ten liver transplant recipients and a liver transplant recipient who underwent autopsy due to primary graft dysfunction. Samples of other possible organs such as the heart, lung, pancreas, and small intestine from this patient were pretreated according to the graft ICFA preparation method. Contaminated blood cells in samples were minimum, confirmed by histology. Luminex analyses detected PE signals from the positive control samples in all organs. Thus, it can be concluded that graft ICFA can be applied for all organ transplantation (**Figure 7**).

3.5. Sensitivity and specificity of graft ICFA to determine pathological AMR in renal transplantation

In order to prove a hypothesis—graft ICFA is useful to detect g-DSA and AMR—a total of 40 Japanese renal transplant recipients were included prospectively. They underwent graft biopsy and were examined by graft ICFA as previously described [19, 20]. According to the results of graft ICFA, these patients were divided into the g-DSA+ and g-DSA- groups to assess

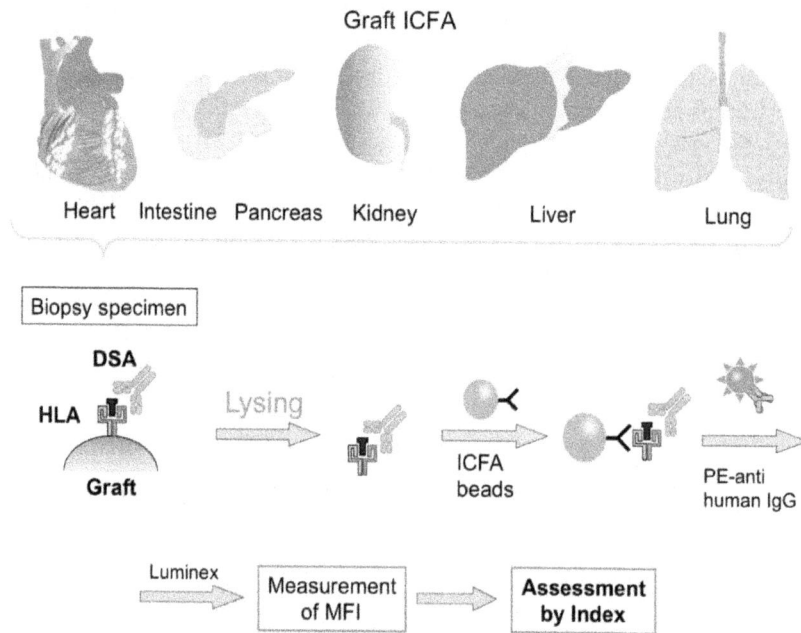

Figure 7. Intra-graft DSA (g-DSA) in all possible allografts can be analyzed by graft ICFA.

the sensitivity and specificity of graft ICFA to predict pathological AMR. In the current study, this technique has demonstrated 100% sensitivity (12/12) and 92.9% specificity (26/28). Thus, it is reasonable to believe that positive graft ICFA results strongly suggest the onset of AMR.

4. Diagnosis of antibody-mediated rejection

4.1. Renal transplantation

With renal allograft dysfunction, it can be diagnosed as AMR, provided that C4d deposited in peritubular capillaries (ptc) and antibodies or complement deposition are confirmed in vascular fibrinoid necrosis, in addition to s-DSA detection. Recently, AMR can be diagnosed according to the Banff classification 2015 [21].

Acute AMR:

The following three criteria should be met when acute AMR is diagnosed:

1. Histological features of acute tissue injury, including at least one of the following

   - Microvascular inflammation g > 0 (excluding recurrent or de novo glomerulonephritis), ptc > 0, or v > 0 (intimal/transmural arteritis).

   - Acute thrombotic microangiopathy (without any other apparent reasons).

   - Acute tubular injury (without any other apparent reasons).

2. Histological features due to DSA and vascular endothelium reaction

   - Linear C4d deposition in ptc (C4d2 or C4d3 (frozen sections)/C4d > 0 (paraffin embedded sections))

   - Moderate microvascular inflammation g + ptc ≥ 2.

   - Detection of genetic transcript expression in biopsy specimens due to endothelial injury.

3. Detection of s-DSA

Chronic AMR:

The following three criteria have to be met:

1. Histological features of chronic tissue injury, including at least one of the following

   - Transplant glomerulopathy (cg > 0), in the case of no chronic thrombotic microangiopathy, includes histologic features detected by electron microscope (EM).

   - Severe ptc basement membrane multilayering by EM.

   - New onset of arterial intimal fibrosis (without any other apparent reasons).

2. Histological features due to DSA and vascular endothelium reaction

- Linear C4d deposition in PTC (C4d2 or C4d3(frozen sections)/C4d > 0 (paraffin embedded sections))

- Moderate microvascular inflammation g + ptc ≥ 2.

- Detection of genetic transcript expression in biopsy specimens due to endothelial injury.

3. Detection of serum DSA

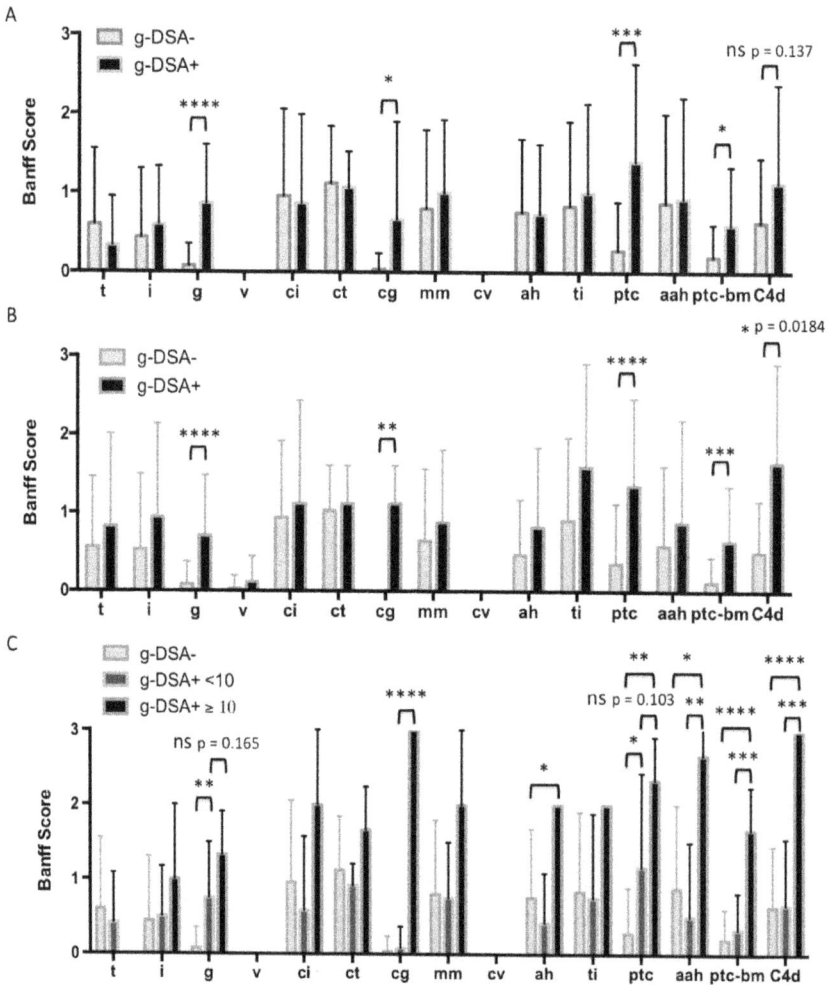

Figure 8. Histopathological impacts of g-DSA presence. A. The Banff histologic scores are analyzed individually based on the g-DSA status: G-DSA- or g-DSA+. B. The Banff histologic scores based on the g-DSA status: G-DSA- or g-DSA+ without ABO-incompatible cases. C. These items are reanalyzed depending on g-DSA values: G-DSA-, g-DSA < 10, and g-DSA ≥ 10, including ABO-incompatible cases. ****p < 0.0001, ***p < 0.0005, **p < 0.005, and *p < 0.05.

4.1.1. The presence of g-DSA (graft ICFA) is associated with microvascular lesions in renal transplantation

To confirm the consistency of graft ICFA results, the individual scores of the Banff classification were analyzed between g-DSA- and g-DSA+ renal transplant recipients (g-DSA+ 15, g-DSA- 25 recipients). As a result, individual g, cg, ptc, and ptc-bm scores were significantly higher in g-DSA+ patients. Interestingly, there was no apparent difference in the C4d staining score, primarily due to the presence of ABO-incompatible cases in both groups (32.0% and 33.3% in the g-DSA- and + groups, respectively) (**Figure 8A**). Thus, ABO-incompatible cases were removed from both groups. Then, the C4d result showed that 0.45 ± 0.17 and 1.73 ± 0.33 in the g-DSA- and g-DSA+ groups, respectively (p = 0.0184) (**Figure 8B**). Next, g-DSA+ patients were divided into low g-DSA group, g-DSA+ < 10, and high g-DSA group, g-DSA+ ≥ 10. Then, this result demonstrated that g and ptc deteriorated in g-DSA concentration manner. In contrast, only g-DSA+ ≥ 10 group showed significant higher scores in cg, mm, ptc-bm, and C4d (**Figure 8C**). These results might indicate that g-DSA causes microcirculation lesions and high g-DSA means chronic allograft damages. To correspond to a recent functional concept, g + ptc (microvascular inflammation), g + cg + ptc (microvascular lesions), and cg + mm (microvascular deterioration), we also analyzed these scores again. Expectedly, g + ptc and g + cg + ptc deteriorated stepwise according to g-DSA scores, but cg + mm referring chronic lesions is clearly higher only in the g-DSA ≥ 10 group (**Figure 9**). It is true, therefore, that g-DSA assessment by graft ICFA accurately supports the diagnosis of AMR.

4.2. Liver transplantation

Generally, it is often discussed that liver allografts tend to be resistant against AMR due to Kupffer cell DSA clearance, HLA expression in microvasculature, allografts size, and regenerative capacity of the liver. Diagnosis criteria are suggested in the Banff meeting [22].

Define acute AMR:

The following four criteria should be met to diagnose acute AMR:

1. Histological features of acute tissue injury, including at least one of the following

   Portal microvascular endothelial cell hypertrophy, eosinophilic and neutrophilic portal microvasculitis, portal edema, and ductular reaction; cholestasis is usually present but variable; edema and periportal hepatocyte necrosis, active lymphocytic, and/or necrotizing arteritis.

2. Positive s-DSA.

3. Diffuse microvascular C4d staining (C4d = 3).

4. Excluding other lesions possibly mimic AMR.

Suspicious for AMR (both criteria required).

Serum DSA + and positive histopathology score (h-score) (C4d + h-score ≥ 3).

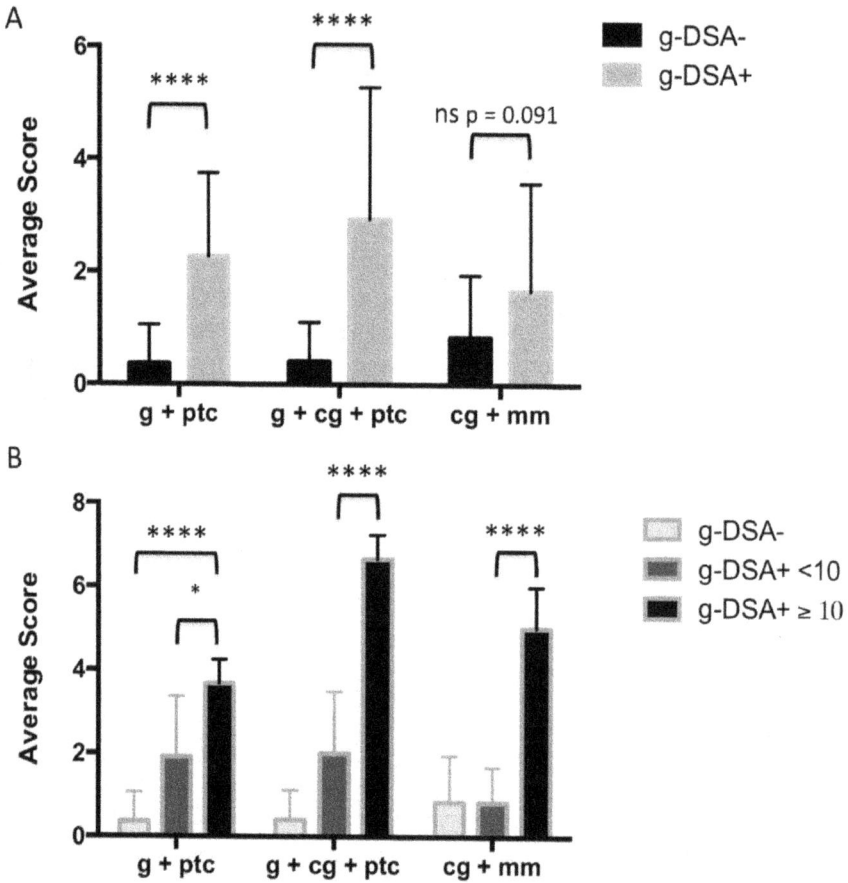

Figure 9. G-DSA effects on the functional clusters of the Banff classification. The functional clusters, g + ptc (microvascular inflammation), g + cg + ptc (microvascular lesions), and cg + mm (microvascular deterioration), are analyzed according to the presence or absence of g-DSA (A) and g-DSA values: G-DSA-, g-DSA < 10, and g-DSA ≥ 10 (B). ****$p < 0.0001$ and *$p < 0.05$.

Indeterminate for AMR:

1. C4d + h-score ≥ 2.

2. DSA and C4d immunohistochemistry not available and not apparent.

3. Coexisting pathophysiology might cause similar injury.

Liver allograft chronic active AMR is also considered as an important factor for determining long-term outcome [23, 24]. Chronic active AMR is diagnosed when the condition meets the all following criteria:

1. Histologic features consistent with chronic active AMR. (a) At least mild mononuclear portal and/or perivenular inflammation with interface and/or perivenular necroinflammatory activity. (b) At least portal/periportal, sinusoidal, and/or perivenular fibrosis.

2. Detection of serum DSA.

3. Focal C4d deposition in portal tract microvascular endothelia (> 10%).

4. Other lesions can be denied.

4.3. Heart transplantation

Following heart transplantation, the onset of AMR is generally estimated around 10–20% [25]. In the field of heart transplantation, AMR is also considered as an important prognosis factor. In fact, the consequences are severe, and the development of cardiac allograft vasculopathy (CAV) has a huge impact. As with other organ transplantations, timing of AMR onset is diverse: both acute AMR within 1 week after transplantation and chronic AMR in the remote period can be seen. Again, allograft biopsy also plays a crucial role to accurately diagnose AMR. Repeated allograft biopsies seem to be required for achieving good long-term outcomes. Interestingly, regarding de novo DSA synthesized after 2 months following heart transplantation, class II DSA are dominant [25].

Diagnosis criteria of heart allograft AMR were discussed in the international society for heart and lung transplantation working formulation consensus [26]. First of all, substrates were divided into two categories: histologic investigations (H) and immunopathologic studies (I). Histologic features of heart AMR are as follows: activated mononuclear cell infiltration, interstitial edema, hemorrhage, necrosis, and vascular thrombosis. On the other hand, C4d, CD68 (paraffin section), C4d, or C3d (frozen section) are considered mandatory panels of immunopathologic studies. Furthermore, CD3, CD20, C3d, endothelial cell CD31 or CD34, complement regulatory proteins (paraffin section), and fibrin and immunoglobulin G/M (frozen section) are regarded as secondary or optional panels. In total, the current report of AMR in heart is noted from Grade 0 to 3 as follows:

pAMR 0: negative for pathologic AMR (H0/I0)

pAMR 1(H+): histopathologic AMR (H+/I−)

pAMR 1 (I+): immunopathologic AMR (H−/I+)

pAMR 2: pathologic AMR (H+/I+)

pAMR 3: severe AMR (interstitial hemorrhage, capillary fragmentation, mixed inflammatory cell infiltration, endothelial cell pyknosis and/or karyorrhexis, and marked edema and I+)

pAMR 3 cases usually demonstrate severe hemodynamic dysfunction and poor consequences.

Scoring system of criteria for pathologic diagnosis of cardiac AMR is slightly different between immunohistochemistry and immunofluorescence analyses. These criteria are summarized in **Table 1**.

4.4. Lung transplantation

Regarding AMR following lung transplantation, the main reason is also DSA, although a role of non-HLA antibodies was also described [27]. Hachem et al. [28] have reported, in 2010, a prospective study on AMR after lung transplantation, which deepened our

Immunohistochemistry scoring system				Immunofluorescence scoring system			
Capillary C4d distribution	0	< 10%	Negative	Capillary C4d/C3d distribution	0	< 10%	Negative
	1	10–50%	Focal		1	10–50%	Focal
	2	> 50%	multifocal/diffuse		2	> 50%	Multifocal/diffuse
Capillary C4d intensity	0	Negative/equivocal		Capillary C4d/C3d intensity	0	Negative/equivocal	
	1	Faint positive			1	Faint positive = 0–1+	
	2	Strong positive			2	Strong positive = 2–3+	
Intravascular CD68 distribution	0	< 10%	Negative	HLA-DR distribution	0	< 10%	Negative
	1	10–50%	Focal		1	10–50%	Focal
	2	> 50%	Multifocal/diffuse		2	> 50%	Multifocal/diffuse
				HLA-DR intensity	0	Negative/equivocal	
					1	Faint positive = 0–1+	
					2	Strong positive = 2–3+	

Table 1. Immunohistochemistry and immunofluorescence scoring system in heart AMR.

understanding of clinical AMR managements. In 2016, a consensus statement has been proposed from the international society for heart and lung transplantation [29].

Lung allograft AMR can be divided into clinical and subclinical AMR, depending on whether there is allograft dysfunction or not. Next, as similar to other organs, these clinical and subclinical AMR are subcategorized as define, probable, or possible. To determine certainty of clinical AMR, the following five criteria are proposed: allograft dysfunction, other causes excluded, lung histology, lung biopsy C4d, and s-DSA. Define lung AMR is determined by positive for all five criteria. In case anyone of them is negative, it is considered as probable AMR, excluding allograft dysfunction (**Table 2**). There are histopathologic features of AMR, including the following—neutrophil margination, neutrophil capillaritis/arteritis without any signs of pneumonia, or other apparent reasons—though these features are not specific for lung AMR. In terms of lung histology, further advancement and organization would be required.

4.5. Small bowel transplantation

Due to recent increased recognition of AMR, AMR is also considered as a serious issue in the small bowel transplantation field. However, the define diagnosis criteria have not been established in the small bowel transplantation yet. There are few series of case reports in terms of intestine AMR. Although common understandings of AMR also seem to be C4d deposition, capillaritis, and s-DSA positivity [30], there is a report which did not find clinical evidence between C4d positivity and the onset of AMR [31]. The establishment of diagnostic criteria should be required to standardize and manage AMR in intestine transplantation. The future contribution of g-DSA assessment would be also expected in this field.

	Allograft dysfunction	Other causes excluded	Lung histology compatible with AMR	C4d	s-DSA
Define	+	+	+	+	+
Probable*	+	+	+	−	+
	+	−	+	+	+
	+	+	−	+	+
	+	+	+	+	−
Possible	+	−	−	+	+
	+	+	−	−	+
	+	+	+	−	−
	+	−	+	−	+
	+	−	+	+	−
	+	+	−	+	−

There is growing evidence that C4d negative AMR exists. Thus, the second line * cases are considered as an independent group.

Table 2. Lung AMR diagnosis criteria.

5. Preoperative desensitization

To perform organ transplantation between a sensitized recipient and donor pair, preoperative desensitization is required. Generally, crossmatch positive organ transplantation is mainly performed in kidney and liver transplantation. Desensitization can be divided into three main treatments: depletion/modification of B cells, apheresis for antibodies, and inhibition of reaction between DSA and HLA. The golden standard of B-cell depletion therapy is rituximab (anti-CD20 antibodies) administration [32–35]. There are a wide variety of rituximab administration protocols in terms of a dosage and schedule. In our institution, generally, rituximab (375 mg/m^2) is administered in 2 weeks prior to organ transplantation [20]. Subsequent B-cell count in the peripheral blood is measured by flow cytometry. In addition to rituximab, to deplete B cells, anti-CD52 antibodies (alemtuzumab) also can be used, because higher than 95% B cells express CD52 on the cell surface [36]. It has been reported that alemtuzumab-combined regimens are safe and effective for highly sensitized recipients [36, 37]. Other antibodies' introduction would be expected regarding induction regimens.

To decrease DSA production and reaction, the importance of intravenous immune globulin (IVIG) has been reported. IVIG infusion significantly decreased the baseline flowPRA levels [38]. There is a variety of reports regarding the dosage and duration of IVIG (100 mg/kg/day–4 g/kg/day, etc.), partially due to the cost problems.

Regarding apheresis therapy, double filtration plasmapheresis (DFPP) or plasma exchange (PE) is generally performed. Usually, as an index of DSA titer, MFI has gained its popularity. Given the fact of g-DSA and s-DSA assessments, DSA with MFI < 2500 might not deposit and cause clinical damages to allografts. Thus, although it depends on each institution, acceptable DSA MFI prior to surgery might be estimated around 2000 [20] in renal transplantation. However, on the other hand, intensive posttransplant desensitization also can result in comparable outcomes with non-sensitized transplantation [39]. For highly sensitized recipients, a phased desensitization protocol by using rituximab and bortezomib was advocated [34]. In fact, it is true that rituximab administration can deplete B cells but not plasma cells. Thus, it is reasonable to believe that rituximab and bortezomib combination therapy eradicates the B-cell linage which is potentially associated with AMR.

Furthermore, the idea only relying on MFI might be unrefined. In other words, the quality of DSA is also important to determine the impact of DSA. Regarding the quality, IgG subclasses [1–4, 40] and complement fixing ability [41] seem to be paid attention, considering the severity of subsequent AMR and graft survival.

On the other hand, in liver transplantation, there seems to be no concrete evidence regarding DSA MFI just prior to transplantation. A large amount of hemorrhage during surgery and liver allograft resistance against DSA, etc., might complicate to set a MFI threshold. Nevertheless, Yoshizawa et al. [42] reported that class I DSA MFI > 10,000 has a negative impact on graft survival. Thus, it is important to keep circumstances where allograft injury due to remnant DSA is minimum and additional DSA production inhibited.

6. Treatment for antibody-mediated rejection

In other words, this is a treatment for B cells/plasma cells and DSA and reaction between DSA and HLA. Both for acute AMR and chronic active AMR, generally clinical managements also can be divided into medications and apheresis: steroid pulse, IVIG, Rituximab, etc., and DFPP or PE. In severe cases, it is true that splenectomy has a certain effect on AMR [43]. Regarding treatment for acute AMR, the concepts are the same: depletion of B cells, reduction of DSA, and inhibition of reaction between DSA and HLA. The core agents and methods are summarized in Table. It is true that high-dose steroid administration is effective on all aspects of AMR treatment. There is no fixed data to determine the dosage and duration of steroid pulse therapy. However, generally, 10–100 mg/kg/day equivalent dosage of hydrocorticoid is administered as steroid pulse therapy, depending on the severity of AMR. For depletion of B cells, rituximab, alemtuzumab, or splenectomy is utilized. To reduce DSA, DFPP, or PE, apheresis methods are commonly used in the same way as desensitization. As immunomodulation, IVIG administration also plays an important role in controlling acute AMR. Given the fact of AMR pathogenesis, complement activation should be paid attention. Final tissue injury due to AMR would occur following activation of antibody-induced terminal complement cascade. Albeit limited evidence, it has been reported that eculizumab C5 inhibitor is effective to rescue an AMR allograft [44–47].

Recently, chronic active AMR has been paid strong attention, because this pathologic condition directly deteriorates the long-term graft survival. Despite the recognition of chronic active AMR, diagnostic criteria are only established in kidney [21] and liver transplantation [22]. There seems to be no therapeutic consensus on this condition. Furthermore, it has generally resistance to ordinal AMR managements discussed above [48–50], although limited effectiveness was observed in few studies [51, 52]. Bachelet et al. [50] reported a treatment for chronic active AMR (mean eGFR 30.6 mL/min/1.73 m^2) by utilizing rituximab (375 mg/m^2) and IVIG (1 g/kg/week × 4 weeks). Although serum MFI tends to decrease, there is no difference in

Treatment for chronic active AMR

Author	Organ	Treatment	Schedule	Outcomes
Billing 2012 [51]	Kidney	IVIG; Rit	1 g/kg/week for 4 weeks; 375 mg/m^2 × 1	The treatment reduced or stabilized the progressive loss of transplant function in pediatric patients
Cooper 2014 [49]	Kidney	IVIG	High-dose (5 g/kg) IVIG dosed over 6 months	No clinical treatment benefit
An 2014* [54]	Kidney	IVIG; Rit	400 mg/kg × 4 days; 375 mg/m^2	The treatment delayed CAMR progression
Bachelet 2015 [50]	Kidney	IVIG; Rit	1 g/kg/week for 4 weeks; 375 mg/m^2/week in the first 2 weeks	The treatment did not seem to change the natural history of AMR
Redfield 2016 [55]	Kidney	Dex; IVIG; Rit (PE, Thymoglobulin)	100 mg of Dex; 4 weekly doses 100 mg/kg; 375 mg/m^2 body, or 1000 mg	Better graft survival
Kulkarni 2017 [53]	Kidney	Eculizmab	600 mg/week for 4 weeks followed by 900 mg every 2 weeks for a total of 26 weeks	Better eGFR in patients with C1q positive
Parajuli 2017 [52]	Kidney	Dex; IVIG; Rit	100 mg; 200 mg/kg/2 weeks for 3 weeks; 375 mg/m^2/week	The treatment was effective in reducing DSA and microcirculation inflammation
Ban 2017* [56]	Kidney	IVIG; Rit	400 mg/kg × 4 days; 375 mg/m^2	The treatment reduced the progression of CAMR

*: Reported from the same group.

Table 3. Summary of recent reports on treatments for chronic active antibody-mediated rejection (AMR).

2-year graft survival between the treatment (47%) and without treatment groups (40%). These reports suggest a difficulty in the management for chronic changes in allografts. In addition to acute AMR, eculizumab was also challenged for chronic active AMR. Although there were no notable differences in eGFR between treatment and control groups, C1q-positive recipients demonstrated significant better eGFR than recipients with C1q-negative status [53]. Inhibition of complement-dependent allograft injury would bring benefits on certain population. Recent reports discussing treatment for chronic active AMR are summarized in **Table 3**.

In total, it is of vital importance to prevent from developing into chronic lesions and initiate appropriate treatment in the early stages of AMR, because fully established chronic lesions are irreversible. It is reasonable to believe that these managements lead to improvements of the long-term allograft survival.

7. Conclusion

Under the present circumstances, it is of vital importance to control AMR in advance in order to improve graft survival rate in all fields of organ transplantation. To detect early-stage AMR, clinicians need to be aware of recent advances in DSA analyses, including graft ICFA and an acid elution method to assess intra-graft DSA status. Preoperative desensitization therapies and management plans are decided depending on classes of DSA and s-DSA MFI. Conversely, even in crossmatch-negative cases, there is a possibility that memory B cells might evoke severe AMR 1 week following transplantation. In addition, there might be a discrepancy between s-DSA and g-DSA. It is also true that only relying on s-DSA MFI is difficult to determine appropriate managements. Further research is required for addressing these issues.

Conflict of interest

None.

Abbreviation

AMR   antibody-mediated rejection

DSA   donor-specific antibodies

ICFA   immunocomplex capture fluorescence analysis

LCT   lymphocyte cytotoxic test

FCXM   flow cytometry crossmatch

SAB   single antigen bead assay

MFI   mean fluorescence intensity

g-DSA   intra-graft DSA

s-DSA   serum DSA

ptc   peritubular capillaries

Author details

Tsukasa Nakamura[1]*, Hidetaka Ushigome[1], Takayuki Shirouzu[2] and Norio Yoshimura[1]

*Address all correspondence to: tsukasa@koto.kpu-m.ac.jp

1 Department of Organ Transplantation and General Surgery, Kyoto Prefectural University of Medicine, Kyoto-prefecture, Japan

2 Wakunaga Pharmaceutical Co., Ltd. Molecular Diagnostics Division, Japan

References

[1] Starzl TE, Marchioro TL, Rifkind D, Holmes JH, Rowlands DT Jr, Waddell WR. Factors in successful renal transplantation. Surgery. 1964;56:296-318

[2] Rapaport FT, Dausset J, Legrand L, Barge A, Lawrence HS, Converse JM. Erythrocytes in human transplantation: Effects of pretreatment with ABO group-specific antigens. The Journal of Clinical Investigation. 1968;**47**(10):2206-2216

[3] Paul LC, van Es LA, Riviere GB, Eernisse G, de Graeff J. Blood group B antigen on renal endothelium as the target for rejection in an ABO-incompatible recipient. Transplantation. 1978;**26**(4):268-271

[4] Kashiwagi N, Corman J, Iwatsuki S, Ishikawa M, Fiala JM, Johansen TS, et al. Mixed lymphocyte culture and graft rejection. Surgical Forum. 1973;**24**:345-348

[5] Wagner H, Cone RE. Adjuvant effect of poly(A:U) upon T cell-mediated in vitro cytotoxic allograft responses. Cellular Immunology. 1974;**10**(3):394-403

[6] Todo S, Porter KA, Kam I, Lynch S, Venkataramanan R, DeWolf A, et al. Canine liver transplantation under Nva2-cyclosporine versus cyclosporine. Transplantation. 1986;**41**(3):296-300

[7] Cosimi AB, Burton RC, Colvin RB, Goldstein G, Delmonico FL, LaQuaglia MP, et al. Treatment of acute renal allograft rejection with OKT3 monoclonal antibody. Transplantation. 1981;**32**(6):535-539

[8] Pena JR, Fitzpatrick D, Saidman SL. Complement-dependent cytotoxicity crossmatch. Methods in Molecular Biology (Clifton, NJ). 2013;**1034**:257-283

[9] Patel R, Terasaki PI. Significance of the positive crossmatch test in kidney transplantation. The New England Journal of Medicine. 1969;**280**(14):735-739

[10] Maguire O, Tario JD Jr, Shanahan TC, Wallace PK, Minderman H. Flow cytometry and solid organ transplantation: A perfect match. Immunological Investigations. 2014;**43**(8):756-774

[11] Nishimura K, Hashimoto M, Kinoshita T, Shiraishi Y, Ueda N, Nakazawa S, et al. Excellent results of immunocomplex capture fluorescence analysis-I for cross-match test in renal transplantation. Transplantation Proceedings. 2014;**46**(2):332-335

[12] Fujiwara K, Shimano K, Tanaka H, Sekine M, Kashiwase K, Uchikawa M, et al. Application of bead array technology to simultaneous detection of human leucocyte antigen and human platelet antigen antibodies. Vox Sanguinis. 2009;**96**(3):244-251

[13] Bray RA, Tarsitani C, Gebel HM, Lee JH. Clinical cytometry and progress in HLA antibody detection. Methods in Cell Biology. 2011;**103**:285-310

[14] Bachelet T, Couzi L, Lepreux S, Legeret M, Pariscoat G, Guidicelli G, et al. Kidney intragraft donor-specific antibodies as determinant of antibody-mediated lesions and poor graft outcome. American Journal of Transplantation : Official Journal of the American Society of Transplantation and the American Society of Transplant Surgeons. 2013;**13**(11):2855-2864

[15] Milongo D, Kamar N, Del Bello A, Guilbeau-Frugier C, Sallusto F, Esposito L, et al. Allelic and Epitopic characterization of intra-kidney allograft anti-HLA antibodies at allograft nephrectomy. American Journal of Transplantation : Official Journal of the American Society of Transplantation and the American Society of Transplant Surgeons. 2016

[16] Nocera A, Tagliamacco A, Cioni M, Innocente A, Fontana I, Barbano G, et al. Kidney Intragraft homing of De novo donor-specific HLA antibodies is an essential step of antibody-mediated damage but not per se predictive of graft loss. American Journal of Transplantation: Official Journal of the American Society of Transplantation and the American Society of Transplant Surgeons. 2017;**17**(3):692-702

[17] Neau-Cransac M, Le Bail B, Guidicelli G, Visentin J, Moreau K, Quinart A, et al. Evolution of serum and intra-graft donor-specific anti-HLA antibodies in a patient with two consecutive liver transplantations. Transplant Immunology. 2015;**33**(2):58-62

[18] Visentin J, Chartier A, Massara L, Linares G, Guidicelli G, Blanchard E, et al. Lung intragraft donor-specific antibodies as a risk factor for graft loss. The Journal of Heart and Lung Transplantation: The Official Publication of the International Society for Heart Transplantation. 2016;**35**(12):1418-1426

[19] Nakamura T, Ushigome H, Watabe K, Imanishi Y, Masuda K, Matsuyama T, et al. Graft Immunocomplex capture fluorescence analysis to detect donor-specific antibodies and HLA antigen complexes in the allograft. Immunological Investigations. 2017;**46**(3):295-304

[20] Nakamura T, Ushigome H, Watabe K, Imanishi Y, Masuda K, Matsuyama T, et al. Influences of pre-formed donor-specific anti-human leukocyte antigen antibodies in living-donor renal transplantation: Results with graft Immunocomplex capture fluorescence analysis. Transplantation Proceedings. 2017;**49**(5):955-958

[21] Loupy A, Haas M, Solez K, Racusen L, Glotz D, Seron D, et al. The Banff 2015 kidney meeting report: Current challenges in rejection classification and prospects for adopting molecular pathology. American Journal of Transplantation : Official Journal of the American Society of Transplantation and the American Society of Transplant Surgeons. 2017;**17**(1):28-41

[22] Demetris AJ, Bellamy C, Hubscher SG, O'Leary J, Randhawa PS, Feng S, et al. Comprehensive update of the Banff working group on liver allograft pathology: Introduction of antibody-mediated rejection. American Journal of Transplantation : Official Journal of the American Society of Transplantation and the American Society of Transplant Surgeons. 2016

[23] Del Bello A, Congy-Jolivet N, Muscari F, Lavayssiere L, Esposito L, Cardeau-Desangles I, et al. Prevalence, incidence and risk factors for donor-specific anti-HLA antibodies in maintenance liver transplant patients. American Journal of Transplantation : Official Journal of the American Society of Transplantation and the American Society of Transplant Surgeons. 2014;**14**(4):867-875

[24] O'Leary JG, Cai J, Freeman R, Banuelos N, Hart B, Johnson M, et al. Proposed diagnostic criteria for chronic antibody-mediated rejection in liver allografts. American Journal of Transplantation: Official Journal of the American Society of Transplantation and the American Society of Transplant Surgeons. 2016;**16**(2):603-614

[25] Kobashigawa J, Crespo-Leiro MG, Ensminger SM, Reichenspurner H, Angelini A, Berry G, et al. Report from a consensus conference on antibody-mediated rejection in heart

transplantation. The Journal of Heart and Lung Transplantation: The Official Publication of the International Society for Heart Transplantation. 2011;**30**(3):252-269

[26] Berry GJ, Burke MM, Andersen C, Bruneval P, Fedrigo M, Fishbein MC, et al. The 2013 International Society for Heart and Lung Transplantation working formulation for the standardization of nomenclature in the pathologic diagnosis of antibody-mediated rejection in heart transplantation. The Journal of Heart and Lung Transplantation: The Official Publication of the International Society for Heart Transplantation. 2013;**32**(12):1147-1162

[27] Shilling RA, Wilkes DS. Immunobiology of chronic lung allograft dysfunction: New insights from the bench and beyond. American Journal of Transplantation : Official Journal of the American Society of Transplantation and the American Society of Transplant Surgeons. 2009;**9**(8):1714-1718

[28] Hachem RR, Yusen RD, Meyers BF, Aloush AA, Mohanakumar T, Patterson GA, et al. Anti-human leukocyte antigen antibodies and preemptive antibody-directed therapy after lung transplantation. The Journal of Heart and Lung Transplantation: The Official Publication of the International Society for Heart Transplantation. 2010;**29**(9):973-980

[29] Levine DJ, Glanville AR, Aboyoun C, Belperio J, Benden C, Berry GJ, et al. Antibody-mediated rejection of the lung: A consensus report of the International Society for Heart and Lung Transplantation. The Journal of Heart and Lung Transplantation: The Official Publication of the International Society for Heart Transplantation. 2016;**35**(4):397-406

[30] Rabant M, Racape M, Petit LM, Taupin JL, Aubert O, Bruneau J, et al. Antibody-mediated rejection in pediatric small bowel transplantation: Capillaritis is a major determinant of C4d positivity in intestinal transplant biopsies. American Journal of Transplantation: Official Journal of the American Society of Transplantation and the American Society of Transplant Surgeons. 2018

[31] de Serre NP, Canioni D, Lacaille F, Talbotec C, Dion D, Brousse N, et al. Evaluation of c4d deposition and circulating antibody in small bowel transplantation. American Journal of Transplantation: Official Journal of the American Society of Transplantation and the American Society of Transplant Surgeons. 2008;**8**(6):1290-1296

[32] Nakao T, Ushigome H, Kawai K, Nakamura T, Harada S, Koshino K, et al. Evaluation of rituximab dosage for ABO-incompatible living-donor kidney transplantation. Transplantation Proceedings. 2015;**47**(3):644-648

[33] Kubal CA, Mangus RS, Saxena R, Lobashevsky A, Higgins N, Agarwal A, et al. Crossmatch-positive liver transplantation in patients receiving thymoglobulin-rituximab induction. Transplantation. 2014;**97**(1):56-63

[34] Ide K, Tanaka Y, Sasaki Y, Tahara H, Ohira M, Ishiyama K, et al. A phased desensitization protocol with rituximab and Bortezomib for highly sensitized kidney transplant candidates. Transplantation Direct. 2015;**1**(5):e17

[35] Ishida H, Furusawa M, Shimizu T, Nozaki T, Tanabe K. Influence of preoperative anti-HLA antibodies on short- and long-term graft survival in recipients with or without rituximab treatment. Transplant International: Official Journal of the European Society for Organ Transplantation. 2014;**27**(4):371-382

[36] Vo AA, Wechsler EA, Wang J, Peng A, Toyoda M, Lukovsky M, et al. Analysis of subcutaneous (SQ) alemtuzumab induction therapy in highly sensitized patients desensitized with IVIG and rituximab. American Journal of Transplantation : Official Journal of the American Society of Transplantation and the American Society of Transplant Surgeons. 2008;8(1):144-149

[37] Kim IK, Choi J, Vo AA, Kang A, Patel M, Toyoda M, et al. Safety and efficacy of Alemtuzumab induction in highly sensitized pediatric renal transplant recipients. Transplantation. 2017;101(4):883-889

[38] Jordan SC, Tyan D, Stablein D, McIntosh M, Rose S, Vo A, et al. Evaluation of intravenous immunoglobulin as an agent to lower allosensitization and improve transplantation in highly sensitized adult patients with end-stage renal disease: Report of the NIH IG02 trial. Journal of the American Society of Nephrology: JASN. 2004;15(12):3256-3262

[39] Amrouche L, Aubert O, Suberbielle C, Rabant M, Van Huyen JD, Martinez F, et al. Long-term outcomes of kidney transplantation in patients with high levels of preformed DSA: The Necker high-risk transplant program. Transplantation. 2017;101(10):2440-2448

[40] Lefaucheur C, Viglietti D, Bentlejewski C. Duong van Huyen JP, Vernerey D, Aubert O, et al. IgG donor-specific anti-human HLA antibody subclasses and kidney allograft antibody-mediated injury. Journal of the American Society of Nephrology: JASN. 2016; 27(1):293-304

[41] Yabu JM, Higgins JP, Chen G, Sequeira F, Busque S, Tyan DB. C1q-fixing human leukocyte antigen antibodies are specific for predicting transplant glomerulopathy and late graft failure after kidney transplantation. Transplantation. 2011;91(3):342-347

[42] Yoshizawa A, Egawa H, Yurugi K, Hishida R, Tsuji H, Ashihara E, et al. Significance of semiquantitative assessment of preformed donor-specific antibody using luminex single bead assay in living related liver transplantation. Clinical & Developmental Immunology. 2013;2013:972705

[43] Locke JE, Zachary AA, Haas M, Melancon JK, Warren DS, Simpkins CE, et al. The utility of splenectomy as rescue treatment for severe acute antibody mediated rejection. American Journal of Transplantation : Official Journal of the American Society of Transplantation and the American Society of Transplant Surgeons. 2007;7(4):842-846

[44] Orandi BJ, Zachary AA, Dagher NN, Bagnasco SM, Garonzik-Wang JM, Van Arendonk KJ, et al. Eculizumab and splenectomy as salvage therapy for severe antibody-mediated rejection after HLA-incompatible kidney transplantation. Transplantation. 2014;98(8): 857-863

[45] Fan J, Tryphonopoulos P, Tekin A, Nishida S, Selvaggi G, Amador A, et al. Eculizumab salvage therapy for antibody-mediated rejection in a desensitization-resistant intestinal re-transplant patient. American Journal of Transplantation : Official Journal of the American Society of Transplantation and the American Society of Transplant Surgeons. 2015;15(7):1995-2000

[46] Thrush PT, Pahl E, Naftel DC, Pruitt E, Everitt MD, Missler H, et al. A multi-institutional evaluation of antibody-mediated rejection utilizing the pediatric heart transplant

study database: Incidence, therapies and outcomes. The Journal of Heart and Lung Transplantation: The Official Publication of the International Society for Heart Transplantation. 2016;**35**(12):1497-1504

[47] Muller YD, Aubert JD, Vionnet J, Rotman S, Sadallah S, Aubert V, et al. Acute antibody-mediated rejection one week after lung transplantation successfully treated with eculizumab, intravenous immunoglobulins and rituximab. Transplantation. 2018

[48] Moreso F, Crespo M, Ruiz JC, Torres A, Gutierrez-Dalmau A, Osuna A, et al. Treatment of chronic antibody mediated rejection with intravenous immunoglobulins and rituximab: A multicenter, prospective, randomized, double-blind clinical trial. American Journal of Transplantation: Official Journal of the American Society of Transplantation and the American Society of Transplant Surgeons. 2018;**18**(4):927-935

[49] Cooper JE, Gralla J, Klem P, Chan L, Wiseman AC. High dose intravenous immunoglobulin therapy for donor-specific antibodies in kidney transplant recipients with acute and chronic graft dysfunction. Transplantation. 2014;**97**(12):1253-1259

[50] Bachelet T, Nodimar C, Taupin JL, Lepreux S, Moreau K, Morel D, et al. Intravenous immunoglobulins and rituximab therapy for severe transplant glomerulopathy in chronic antibody-mediated rejection: A pilot study. Clinical Transplantation. 2015;**29**(5):439-446

[51] Billing H, Rieger S, Susal C, Waldherr R, Opelz G, Wuhl E, et al. IVIG and rituximab for treatment of chronic antibody-mediated rejection: A prospective study in paediatric renal transplantation with a 2-year follow-up. Transplant International: Official Journal of the European Society for Organ Transplantation. 2012;**25**(11):1165-1173

[52] Parajuli S, Mandelbrot DA, Muth B, Mohamed M, Garg N, Aziz F, et al. Rituximab and monitoring strategies for late antibody-mediated rejection after kidney transplantation. Transplantation Direct. 2017;**3**(12):e227

[53] Kulkarni S, Kirkiles-Smith NC, Deng YH, Formica RN, Moeckel G, Broecker V, et al. Eculizumab therapy for chronic antibody-mediated injury in kidney transplant recipients: A pilot randomized controlled trial. American Journal of Transplantation: Official Journal of the American Society of Transplantation and the American Society of Transplant Surgeons. 2017;**17**(3):682-691

[54] An GH, Yun J, Hong YA, Khvan M, Chung BH, Choi BS, et al. The effect of combination therapy with rituximab and intravenous immunoglobulin on the progression of chronic antibody mediated rejection in renal transplant recipients. Journal of Immunology Research. 2014;**2014**:828732

[55] Redfield RR, Ellis TM, Zhong W, Scalea JR, Zens TJ, Mandelbrot D, et al. Current outcomes of chronic active antibody mediated rejection - a large single center retrospective review using the updated BANFF 2013 criteria. Human Immunology. 2016

[56] Ban TH, Yu JH, Chung BH, Choi BS, Park CW, Kim YS, et al. Clinical outcome of rituximab and intravenous immunoglobulin combination therapy in kidney transplant recipients with chronic active antibody-mediated rejection. Annals of Transplantation: Quarterly of the Polish Transplantation Society. 2017;**22**:468-474

Chapter 4

HLA Class II Allele Polymorphisms and the Clinical Outcomes of HBV Infection

Shuyun Zhang

Additional information is available at the end of the chapter

http://dx.doi.org/10.5772/intechopen.81366

Abstract

In 2016, the global health sector strategy (GHSS) on viral hepatitis called for elimination of hepatitis B as a major public health threat by 2030 (i.e., 90% reduction in incidence and 65% in mortality). But persistence or clearance of hepatitis B virus (HBV) infection mainly depends upon host immune responses. The human leukocyte antigen (HLA) system is the center of host immune responses. HLA genes are located in chromosome 6p21.31 and cover 0.13% of the human genome and show a high degree of polymorphism and extensive patterns of linkage disequilibrium (LD), which differ among populations. The HLA genes include HLA class I, HLA class II, and other non-HLA alleles. HLA class II gene polymorphisms are strongly associated with not only persistent HBV infection but also spontaneous HBV clearance and seroconversion, disease progression, and the development of liver cirrhosis (LC) and HBV-related hepatocellular carcinoma (HCC) in chronic hepatitis B. This chapter summarizes the reported associations of HLA class II gene polymorphisms with the outcomes of HBV infection and their related mechanisms.

Keywords: HBV, HBV infection, HLA, HLA class II gene polymorphisms

1. Introduction

Since the discovery of hepatitis B virus (HBV) by Blumberg et al. in 1965, much has been elucidated regarding its virion, infection, prevention, and treatment [1, 2]. However, HBV infection continues to be a significant public health problem that has not yet been fully addressed worldwide [3, 4].

HBV infection is caused by HBV, an enveloped DNA virus that infects the liver causing hepatocellular inflammation and necrosis. HBV infection can be either acute or chronic, and the associated illness ranges in severity from asymptomatic to symptomatic and progressive disease. Chronic hepatitis B (CHB) is defined as persistence of hepatitis B surface antigen (HBsAg) for 6 months or more [2]. The World Health Organization (WHO) reports that 80–90% of infants infected during the first year of life and 30–50% of children infected before the age of 6 years develop chronic infections; less than 5% of otherwise healthy persons who are infected as adults will develop chronic infection; and 20–30% of adults who are chronically infected will develop cirrhosis and/or liver cancer [4]. In 2015, 257 million people lived with HBV infection defined as hepatitis B surface antigen positive; and hepatitis B resulted in 887,000 deaths, mostly from complications including liver cirrhosis (LC) and hepatocellular carcinoma (HCC) [4]. Once infected with HBV, one of the main risks is the development of cirrhosis, hepatic decompensation, and ultimately HCC [2–6]. In 2016, the global health sector strategy (GHSS) on viral hepatitis called for elimination of viral hepatitis as a major public health threat by 2030 (i.e., 90% reduction in incidence and 65% in mortality) [5]. In 2017, WHO's first-ever Global hepatitis report presented the baseline values for each of the core indicators of the strategy [6].

The prevention component of elimination is on track with respect to hepatitis B vaccination, blood safety, and injection safety [7–10]. A promising but limited start in hepatitis testing and treatment needs to be followed by immediate and sustained action so that we reach the service coverage targets required to achieve elimination by 2030 [3]. Levrero et al. [11], Vyas et al. [12], and Yoo et al. [13] reviewed that multiple emerging drug therapies are currently in the early stages of development as part of the growing effort to find a true cure for HBV. But persistence or clearance of HBV infection mainly depends upon host immune responses.

The major histocompatibility complex (MHC) was discovered in the mouse in 1936 [14]. The human leukocyte antigen (HLA) system, MHC in humans, is the center of host immune responses [15–17]. HLA genes are located in chromosome 6p21.31 [18] and cover 0.13% of the human genome [19] and show a high degree of polymorphism and extensive patterns of linkage disequilibrium (LD), which differ among populations. The HLA genes include HLA class I, HLA class II, and other non-HLA alleles [20]. HLA class I alleles include the three classic HLA gene loci: HLA-A, HLA-B, and HLA-C; three non-classic HLA-E, HLA-F, and HLA-G gene loci, which show limited polymorphism compared to the classic class I loci; and other related non-coding genes and pseudogenes [20]. The main function of HLA class I molecules, which are expressed in all nucleated cells, is to present non-self antigens derived from intracellular sources, such as viruses, to CD8$^+$ T cells (cytotoxic T cells, CTL), which then identify and kill infected cells [21]. CD8$^+$ T cells interact with the cognate peptide-MHC I complexes via their T-cell receptor (TCR) and co-receptor molecule CD8. HLA class II alleles include the classic gene loci HLA-DR, HLA-DQ, and HLA-DP and also the non-classic HLA-DO and HLA-DM loci [20]. The classic genes are expressed on the surface of professional antigen-presenting cells (APCs), which take up antigens derived from extracellular sources [22], such as bacteria or food, and present them to CD4$^+$ T helper cells. This leads to the secretion of various small proteins, including cytokines, which regulate other immune cells such as macrophages or B cells. In turn, macrophages can destroy ingested microbes, and activated B cells can secrete antibodies. CD4$^+$ T cells interact with the cognate peptide-MHC II complexes via their TCR and the co-receptor molecule CD4. Non-classic molecules are exposed in internal membranes in lysosomes, which help load antigenic peptides on to classic MHC class II molecules. Over the past 50 years, polymorphisms in the HLA locus have been shown to influence many critical biological traits and individuals' susceptibility to complex, autoimmune, and infectious diseases [17, 23, 24]. Since 1979, Kew et al. [25] started the research for the association between histocompatibility antigens and HBV infection, and a plenty of researches demonstrated that the highly polymorphic HLA classes I and II genes can affect the ability of HLA molecules to trigger immune responses, which affects the outcomes of HBV infection, and discrepant conclusions were reached in different cohorts [26, 27]. HLA class II gene polymorphisms are strongly associated with not only persistent HBV infection but also spontaneous HBV clearance and seroconversion, disease progression, and the development of LC and HBV-related HCC in chronic hepatitis B [28–30]. This chapter summarizes the reported associations of HLA class II gene polymorphisms with susceptibility to HBV infection, resolution, and disease progression and their related mechanisms.

2. HLA class II gene and the clinical outcomes of HBV infection

HLA class II gene includes $HLA-DRA_1$, $-DRB_{1-9}$, $-DQA_1$, $-DQB_1$, $-DPA_1$, $-DPA_2$, $-DPB_1$, $-DPB_2$, -DOA, -DOB, -DMA, and -DMB with 4857 alleles known with the latest report update on April 16, 2018 (http://www.ebi.ac.uk/imgt/hla/stats.html). HLA-DRB1 has the most allelic variability with 2165 alleles, and in turn HLA-DQB1 with 1196 alleles, HLA-DPB1 with 975 alleles, and HLA-DRB3 with 157 alleles [20].

2.1. HLA class II allele polymorphism and HBV infection outcomes

HLA-DR is widely used in transplant gene matching [31] and as an activated T cell surface marker [32], and early related to the clinical outcomes of HBV infection [33]. In 2013, we reviewed the relationship between HLA class II alleles and HBV infection, there are the most number of HLA-DR alleles relatived to HBV infection, such as $HLA-DRB_1$*03, 07, 09 and 12, may be the risk factors of HBV infection; and $HLA-DRB_1$*04, 11, 13 and 14 may be the protect factors of HBV infection [26]. In 2016, Wang et al. also reviewed the relationship of HLA-DR alleles with HBV infection [27], including $HLA-DRB_1$*1301-02 which is consistently associated with HBV clearance globally, such as in Gambia, Germany, Korea, and Spain; $HLA-DRB_1$*11 and $-DRB_1$*14 are associated with spontaneous recovery in patients with HBV subgenotype C2 infection in Northeast China; $HLA-DR_2$, HLA-DR*0406, and $HLA-DR_7$ antigens are associated with protective effect on acute HBV infection; and $HLA-DRB_1$*08 and $-DRB_1$*09 alleles, which are susceptible to HBV infection, were found in Brazilian populations determined in young and male blood donors. Meanwhile, $HLA-DRB_1$*11/12 alleles are associated with HBV persistence globally, and $HLA-DRB_1$*07 is the only one associated with infant susceptibility to intrauterine HBV infection and a significant negative predictor of cirrhosis. Our researches also showed that: $-DRB_1$*13 may protect subjects from HBV infection [26]; $-DRB_1$*12 may have a high risk for HBV infection [26]; and $-DRB_1$*07 and 12 may be implied in viral persistence [26, 34]. Analysis still identified $HLA-DRB_1$*12:02 as the top susceptible HLA allele associated with acute-on-chronic liver failure (ACLF) [35]. A large number of studies have been conducted to identify HLA-DRB1 genetic variants associated with HCC risk and clinical out-comes, but many of the findings in these studies are inconsistent and inconclusive [36–38]. A meta-analysis by Lin et al. reported an ethnicity-dependent association between specific HLA-DRB1 alleles and HCC risk, DRB_1*07 and DRB_1*12 were significantly associated with the risk of HCC in the whole populations, and DRB_1*15 allele significantly increased the risk of hepatocellular carcinoma only in Asians [36]. One research by Ma et al. suggests that if genetic factors play a role in familial aggregation of hepatocellular carcinoma, the defi-ciency in the DRB_1*11 and DRB_1*12 alleles might be the risk factor at work in the Guangxi Zhuang Autonomous Region, P.R.C. [37]. Another meta-analysis by Liu et al. reported that HLA-DRB_1*01 and 11 alleles were protective factors, while HLA-DRB_1*12 and 14 alleles were risk factors for HCC development [38]. These findings are somewhat reasonable considering the incidence and distribution of HCC which are closely linked to environmental, dietary, and lifestyle factors, as well as genetic profiles, but the risk for HCC was not controlled for possible confounders such as HBV or HCV, which are more prone to bias than that of the randomized clinical trial studies.

HLA-DQ belongs to one of HLA class II molecules; it is also expressed as cell-surface glycopro-teins that bind to exogenous antigens and present them to CD4$^+$ T cells. HLA-DQ molecules function as a heterodimer of alpha and beta subunits which are encoded by the HLA-DQA_1 and HLA-DQB_1 genes, respectively. HLA-DQs are highly polymorphic especially in exon 2 which encode antigen-binding sites. Therefore, a number of alleles have been declared to be associated with persistent HBV infection [26, 27] — HLA-DQA_1*0102, 0201, 0301, and 0402 and HLA-DQB_1*0604, and so on associated with HBV clearance; and HLA-DQA_1*0103, 0201, 0302, and 0501 and HLA DQB_1*0301, and so on associated with HBV persistence [26]; the two-locus haplotype consisting of -DQA_1*0501 and -DQB_1*0301, and the three-locus haplotype consisting of -DQA_1*0501, -DQB_1*0301, and -DRB_1*1102 were significantly associated with persistent HBV infection in an African-American cohort; -DQB_1*0301 was associated with HBV persistence globally; in addition, -DQB_1*0201 is a HBV-resistant gene, and -DQB_1*0303 is a susceptibility gene of carrying HBV in Xinjiang Uygur ethnic groups of China; and -DQB_1*0503 are associated with early HBeAg seroconversion in CHB children in Taiwan [27]. HLA genotyping-based analysis identified -DQB_1*0601 as having the strongest association, showing a greater association with CHB susceptibility [28].

The HLA DPA_1 and HLA DPB_1 belong to the HLA class II alpha and beta chain paralogs, which also make a heterodimer consisting of an alpha and a beta chain on the surface of antigen-presenting cells. This HLA class II molecule also plays a central role in the immune system by presenting peptides derived from extracellular proteins. Identification of a total of five alleles, including two risk alleles (DPB_1*09:01 and DPB_1*05:01) and three protective alleles (DPB_1*04:01, DPB_1*04:02, and DPB_1*02:01), would enable HBV-infected individuals to be classified into groups according to the treatment requirements. Moreover, among the five reported HLA-DPB_1 susceptibility alleles, three DPB_1 alleles (DPB_1*05:01, *02:01, and *04:02) had primary effects on CHB susceptibility. However, the association of the remaining two alleles (DPB_1*09:01 and *04:01) had come from LD with HLA-DR-DQ haplotypes (i.e., DRB_1*15:02-DQB_1*06:01 and DRB_1*13:02-DQB_1*06:04, respectively) [28, 39].

2.2. Single nucleotide polymorphisms at HLA class II gene and HBV infection outcomes

HLA gene variations are strongly associated with HBV infection outcomes in not only HLA alleles but also single nucleotide polymorphisms (SNPs) identified through genome-wide associated studies (GWASs). Recent GWASs have revealed several SNPs at HLA class II region associated with the risk of HBV infection [23, 30].

A Chinese study by Zhu et al. [40] identified two HLA-DR loci that independently drive chronic HBV infection, including HLA-DRβ113 sites 71 and rs400488. Acute-on-chronic liver failure (ACLF) is an extreme condition after severe acute exacerbation of chronic hepatitis B. Tan et al. carried out a genome-wide association study, among 1300 ACLFs and 2087 AsCs, and identified rs3129859 at HLA class II region (chromosome 6p21.32) which is associated with HBV-related ACLF. Analysis identified HLA-DRB$_1$*12:02 as the top susceptible HLA allele associated with ACLF. The association of rs3129859 was robust in ACLF subgroups or HBV e antigen-negative chronic hepatitis B phase. Clinical traits analysis in patients with ACLF showed that the risky rs3129859*C allele was also associated with prolonged pro-thrombin time, faster progression to ascites development, and higher 28-day mortality [35]. SNP rs9272105 locates between HLA-DQA$_1$ and HLA-DRB$_1$ on 6p21.32. SNP imputation in the GWAS discovery samples revealed additional SNPs showing association, but rs9272105 remained the top SNP within the region [41], which successfully validated the associations between rs9272105 and HCC risk [42]. Of the 12 SNPs reported in HBV-related HCC GWASs, rs2647073 and rs3997872 near HLA-DRB1 were found to be significantly associated with the risk of HBV-related LC, which suggested that genetic variants associated with HBV-related hepatocarcinogenesis may already play an important role in the progression from CHB to LC [43]. A recent study reported new SNPs at HLA-DRB$_1$ (rs35445101) associated with TP53 expression status in HBV-related hepatocellular carcinoma [30].

In 2013, Jiang et al. first found the association of HCC risk with rs9275319 at 6p21.3 located between HLA-DQB$_1$ and HLA-DQA$_2$, which was not reported in earlier GWASs of HCC [44]. Their following research and that of Wen et al. successfully validated the associations between rs9275319 and HCC risk [42, 43]. Three SNPs belonging to the HLA-DQ region (rs2856718, rs7453920, and rs9275572) were studied. HLA-DQ rs2856718G, rs7453920A, and rs9275572A were strongly associated with decreased risk of chronic HBV infection and natural clearance; while rs2856718A, rs7453920G, and rs9275572G served as a risk factor in HBV infection in Japanese populations and in Southeast China [45–48]. Chang et al. found that rs9276370 (HLA-DQA$_2$), rs7756516, and rs7453920 (HLA-DQB$_2$) are significantly associated with persis-tent HBV infection, especially the "T-T" haplotype composed of rs7756516 and rs9276370 that is more prevalent in severe disease subgroups and associated with nonsustained therapeutic response in male Taiwan Han Chinese individuals [49]. A nearest study reported four new SNPs at HLA-DQB$_1$ (rs1130399, rs1049056, rs1049059, and rs1049060) associated with TP53 expression status in HBV-related HCC [30].

A Chinese study by Zhu et al. [40] identified HLA-DPβ$_1$ positions 84–87 that indepen-dently drive chronic HBV infection. In 2009, Kamatani et al. first reported two SNPs with the strongest relation to HBV infection from the HLA-DP locus: rs3077 on HLA DPA1 and rs9277535 on HLA DPB$_1$ in Japanese and Thai populations [50, 51]. Subsequently, plenty of studies further demonstrated their roles [27, 52–54]. rs3077 and rs9277535 are significantly related to HBV persistent infection and both A alleles of these two SNPs are protection alleles in Chinese Han [55], Japanese and Korean [56], and European [57] populations, while in Chinese Zhuang subjects, only HLA-DP rs9277535A is associated with decreased risk [55]. Also, only a highly significant association of HLA-DPA$_1$ rs3077C with HBV infection was observed in Caucasians [58]. HBeAg-negative HBV carriers with rs9277535 non-GG genotype had a higher chance to clear HBsAg. Compared to GG haplotype of rs3077 and rs9277535, GA haplotype had a higher chance of achieving spontaneous HBsAg loss in Chinese subjects of Taiwan [59]. On the whole, the present findings show that SNPs rs3077 and rs9277535 at HLA-DP locus protect against HBV infection and increase the chance of HBV clearance, while the importance of these polymorphisms as a predictor of HCC may be limited [45, 60, 61]. In a report by Hu et al., HLA-DP rs3077 showed an approaching significant effect on susceptibility to HBV persistent infection and HCC development when considering multiple testing adjustments [62]. Li et al. found evidence for the association at rs9277535 with HCC independently by imputation [41]. Thomas et al. reported that SNPs rs3077 and rs9277535 that associated most significantly with chronic hepatitis B and outcomes of HBV infection in Asians had a marginal effect on HBV recovery in European and African-American samples. However, they identified a novel variant in the HLA-DPB$_1$ 3′UTR region, 496A/G (rs9277534), which associated very significantly with HBV recovery in both European and African-American populations [63]. Hu et al. also found that the variant at rs9277534 could affect both the spontaneous clearance of HBV infection and progression from asymptomatic HBV carriers to HBV-related liver cirrhosis in southwest Han Chinese population [64]. Chang et al. found that rs9366816 near HLA-DPA3 are significantly associated with persistent HBV infection in male Taiwan Han Chinese individuals [49]. A nearest study reported a new SNP at HLA-DPB1 (rs1042153) associated with TP53 expression status in HBV-related hepatocellular carcinoma [30].

2.3. The role and mechanism of HLA class II gene variations associated with HBV infection outcomes

HLA class II genes encode proteins expressed on the surface of antigen-presenting cells such as macrophages, dendritic cells, and B cells, and thereby have a critical role in the presentation of antigens to CD4+ T-helper lymphocytes. In our previous review, there were three mechanisms related to HBV infection outcomes, including HLA molecular structure, HLA gene expression, and its regulatory [26].

HLA class II genes have many structural variants that have been linked to immune response [65, 66] to autoimmune diseases [67, 68], idiosyncratic drug toxicity (IDT) [69, 70], and infectious agents [71, 72]. But the structural variants related to HBV infection outcomes in HLA class II genes only have our previous research report [73]. We know that the HLA class II molecules are heterodimeric glycoproteins, which are able to present peptides to CD4+ T cells; the primary protein sequences (α1 and β1 chains) encoded by the second exon of the HLA class II genes comprise the peptide-binding grooves that accommodate amino acid chains of the bound peptides; the specificity of the peptide-binding grooves is governed by the properties of pockets in the grooves which include nine different structural pockets (Ps) from P1 to P9, typical pockets being P1, P4, P6, and P9, which accommodate the antigen peptide side chains; and the polymorphic residues encoded by polymorphic HLA class II genes can influence the structural (size and shape) and electrostatic properties and further function of the pockets. So, the determination of the structural and electrostatic properties of the HLA class II peptide-binding grooves associated with diseases may help identify the disease mechanism. We found that DR07 and DR12 carry amino acids Leu and His at residue 30 of HLA-DRβ1 chain, respectively, and Val at residue 57 of HLA-DRβ1 chain, difference from Tyr30 and Asp57 carried by DR04 and DR11, leading to present positive charge at P9 [73], as well as increasing size due to the absence of an intact salt bridge at P6 and P9 [73, 74]. Hence, which HLA DR07 and DR12 is sufficient to chronic HBV infection is supported by the structure characters resulting from HLA gene polymorphism.

Gene expression, that is, the qualitative and quantitative expression of mRNA transcripts from DNA templates, forms a first link in the functional path between nucleotide sequence and higher-order organismal phenotypes. Despite the undeniable importance of a controlled gene regulatory process in which proper transcripts are expressed at the correct time and location, studies have shown that there is widespread inter-individual variability with respect to gene expression, or mRNA levels, within a given cell type or tissue [75]. Early in 1986, Edwards et al. [76] examined frozen sections of human fetal spleen from 12 to 20 weeks of gestation by using polyclonal antibodies to Ig isotypes, monoclonal antibodies to HLA class II subregion locus products, B and T cells, and follicular dendritic cells. Their data suggest that class II antigens are differentially expressed on developing lymphoid cells; DR and DP expression occurring in the earliest spleens examined, with expression of DP on a subpopulation of DR-positive cells; IgD and DQ expression appears to be coincident on maturing B cells as they begin to form follicles, and an immunoregulatory role for HLA-DQ in B cell development is implicated. In fact, HLA class II gene (HLA-DR) expression level is still one of the markers for immune reaction related to disease [33, 77]. In 2017, we reviewed the association of HLA-DR expression level with diseases and reported our studies about the characteristics of HLA-DR expression in patients with different outcomes of HBV infection. Compared to persons with no HBV marker, HBV infection and vaccination induce increased expression of HLA-DR, especially in the clearance of HBV infection [78]. Genetic variants that influence HLA mRNA expression might also affect antigen presentation and many "gene expression-associated SNPs" (eSNPs) have been found for HLA genes [79, 80]. An integrated approach combining genotype information with genome-wide gene expression data in relevant tissues can identify genetic variations that are both regulatory and disease causing [81]. Cavalli et al. believed that a majority of causal genetic variants underlying complex diseases appear to involve regulatory elements, rather than coding variations [82]. Kaur et al. reported that structural and regulatory diversity shape HLA-C protein expression levels and that quantitative variation in the expression of *HLA-C* can influence the clinical course of HIV infection and the risk of graft-versus-host disease [83]. By influencing HLA mRNA expression, rs3077 and rs9277535 variants, both are noncoding variation (3'UTR) in the HLA-DPA$_1$ and HLA-DPB$_1$ region, and are related to enhanced clearance of hepatitis B virus infection [57, 63] and increased risk of graft-versus-host disease in mismatched hematopoietic cell transplant recipients [84, 85]. These findings were identified by a study about mapping of hepatic expression quantitative trait loci (eQTLs) in a Han Chinese population by Wang et al. [86].

eQTLs, namely, the discovery of genetic variants, explain variation in gene expression levels which has significant differences in mean expression levels between population, tissue or cell type [75, 87]. Typically, in the eQTL mapping literature, regulatory variants have been characterized as either cis or trans acting, reflecting the predicted nature of interactions and of course depending on the physical distance from the gene they regulate. Conventionally, variants within 1–2 Mb (megabase) on either side of a gene's TSS were called cis, while those at least 5 Mb downstream or upstream of the TSS or on a different chromosome were considered trans acting [87]. The most significant GWAS SNPs are strong eQTLs and proposing candidate disease genes. Multiple variants of low-effect sizes affect multiple genes by gene regulatory network. A network component can be viewed as a cis effect that transmits its signal in trans essentially making the cis SNP a trans SNP as well [87]. Such studies have offered promise not just for the characterization of functional sequence variation but also for the understanding of basic processes of gene regulation and interpretation of genome-wide association studies [75, 87].

Up to now, many research findings have demonstrated that HLA class II gene variations, including allele polymorphisms and SNPs, are associated with HBV infection outcomes by influencing the molecular structure and the expression level of HLA class II molecules expressed on the cell surface. As the researches progress with methodological improvements, such as the prediction of gene expression [88] and PrediXcan analysis [89], more structure variations, cis SNPs and trans SNPs, were found underlying this disease. This can help understand the mechanisms linking genome-wide association loci to the disease, and implement precise individualized prevention, diagnosis, and treatment of the disease.

Acknowledgements

This work was supported by Wu Jieping Medical Foundation [Grant number 320.6750.18230].

Conflict of interest

None.

Author details

Shuyun Zhang

Address all correspondence to: zhang13214501198@163.com

Research Center, The Second Affiliated Hospital of Harbin Medical University, Harbin, Heilongjiang Province, P.R. China

References

[1] Blumberg BS, Alter HJ, Visnich S. A "new" antigen in leukemia sera. Journal of the American Medical Association. 1984;**252**(2):252-257. DOI: 10.1001/jama.1984.03350020054026

[2]   WHO Guidelines Approved by the Guidelines Review Committee. Guidelines for the Prevention, Care and Treatment of Persons with Chronic Hepatitis B Infection. Geneva: World Health Organization; 2015. PMID: 26225396

[3]   Hutin YJ, Bulterys M, Hirnschall GO. How far are we from viral hepatitis elimination service coverage targets? Journal of the International AIDS Society. 2018;21(Suppl 2): e25050. DOI: 10.1002/jia2.25050

[4]   WHO. Hepatitis B. 2017. Available from: New hepatitis data highlight need for urgent global response

[5]   WHO. Global Health Sector Strategy on Viral Hepatitis, 2016-2021. 2016. Available from: http://apps.who.int/iris/bitstream/10665/246177/1/WHO-HIV-2016.06-eng.pdf?ua=1

[6]   WHO. Global Hepatitis Report. 2017. Available from: http://www.who.int/hepatitis/publications/global-hepatitis-report2017/en/ Google Scholar

[7]   Lin CL, Kao JH. Review article: The prevention of hepatitis B-related hepatocellular carcinoma. Alimentary Pharmacology & Therapeutics. 2018;48(1):5-14. DOI: 10.1111/apt.14683

[8]   Tang LSY, Covert E, Wilson E, Kottilil S. Chronic hepatitis B infection: A review. Journal of the American Medical Association. 2018;319(17):1802-1813. DOI: 10.1001/jama.2018.3795

[9]   Duffell EF, Hedrich D, Mardh O, Mozalevskis A. Towards elimination of hepatitis B and C in European Union and European Economic Area countries: Monitoring the World Health Organization's global health sector strategy core indicators and scaling up key interventions. Euro Surveillance. 2017;22(9):pii:30476. DOI: 10.2807/1560-7917.ES.2017.22.9.30476

[10] Stępień M, Zakrzewska K, Rosińska M. Significant proportion of acute hepatitis B in Poland in 2010-2014 attributed to hospital transmission: Combining surveillance and public registries data. BMC Infectious Diseases. 2018;18(1):164. DOI: 10.1186/s12879-018-3063-3

[11] Levrero M, Testoni B, Zoulim F. HBV cure: Why, how, when? Current Opinion in Virology. 2016;18:135-143. DOI: 10.1016/j.coviro.2016.06.003

[12] Vyas AK, Jindal A, Hissar S, Ramakrishna G, Trehanpati N. Immune balance in hepatitis B infection: Present and future therapies. Scandinavian Journal of Immunology. 2017;86(1):4-14. DOI: 10.1111/sji.12553

[13] Yoo J, Hann HW, Coben R, Conn M, DiMarino AJ. Update treatment for HBV infection and persistent risk for hepatocellular carcinoma: Prospect for an HBV cure. Diseases. 2018;6(2):pii:E27. DOI: 10.3390/diseases6020027

[14] Gorer PA. The detection of a hereditary antigenic difference in the blood of mice by means of human group a serum. Journal of Genetics. 1936;32:17-31. DOI: 10.1007/BF02982499

[15] Kelly A, Trowsdale J. Introduction: MHC/KIR and governance of specificity. Immunogenetics. 2017;69(8-9):481-488. DOI: 10.1007/s00251-017-0986-6

[16] Meyer D, C Aguiar VR, Bitarello BD, C Brandt DY, Nunes K. A genomic perspective on HLA evolution. Immunogenetics. 2018;70(1):5-27. DOI: 10.1007/s00251-017-1017-3. Epub 2017 Jul 7

[17] Phillips KP, Cable J, Mohammed RS, Herdegen-Radwan M, Raubic J, Przesmycka KJ, et al. Immunogenetic novelty confers a selective advantage in host-pathogen coevolution. Proceedings of the National Academy of Sciences of the United States of America. 2018;**115**(7):1552-1557. DOI: 10.1073/pnas.1708597115

[18] Singh R, Kaul R, Kaul A, Khan K. A comparative review of HLA associations with hepatitis B and C viral infections across global populations. World Journal of Gastroenterology. 2007;**13**(12):1770-1787. DOI: 10.3748/wjg.v13.i12.1770

[19] Shiina T, Hosomichi K, Inoko H, Kulski JK. The HLA genomic loci map: Expression, interaction, diversity and disease. Journal of Human Genetics. 2009;**54**(1):15-39. DOI: 10.1038/jhg.2008.5

[20] Robinson J, Halliwell JA, Hayhurst JH, Flicek P, Parham P, Marsh SGE. The IPD and IPD-IMGT/HLA database: Allele variant databases. Nucleic Acids Research. 2015;**43**: D423-D431. DOI: 10.1093/nar/gku1161

[21] Bailey A, Dalchau N, Carter R, Emmott S, Phillips A, Werner JM, et al. Selector function of MHC I molecules is determined by protein plasticity. Scientific Reports. 2015;**5**:14928. DOI: 10.1038/srep14928

[22] Holling TM, Schooten E, van Den Elsen PJ. Function and regulation of MHC class II molecules in T-lymphocytes: Of mice and men. Human Immunology. 2004;**65**:282-290. DOI: 10.1016/j.humimm.2004.01.005

[23] Matzaraki V, Kumar V, Wijmenga C, Zhernakova A. The MHC locus and genetic susceptibility to autoimmune and infectious diseases. Genome Biology. 2017;**18**(1):76. DOI: 10.1186/s13059-017-1207-1

[24] Naranbhai V, Carrington M. Host genetic variation and HIV disease: From mapping to mechanism. Immunogenetics. 2017;**69**(8-9):489-498. DOI: 10.1007/s00251-017-1000-z

[25] Kew MC, Gear AJ, Baumgarten I, Dusheiko GM, Maier G. Histocompatibility antigens in patients with hepatocellular carcinoma and their relationship to chronic hepatitis B virus infection in these patients. Gastroenterology. 1979;**77**(3):537-539 222645

[26] Yu XY, Zhang SY. Development of relationship research between human leukocyte antigen and clinical changes of hepatitis B viral infections. Chinese Journal of Infectious Diseases. 2013;**31**(10):635-638

[27] Wang L, Zou ZQ, Wang K. Clinical relevance of HLA gene variants in HBV infection. Journal of Immunology Research. 2016;**2016**:9069375. DOI: 10.1155/2016/9069375

[28] Nishida N, Ohashi J, Khor SS, Sugiyama M, Tsuchiura T, Sawai H, et al. Understanding of HLA-conferred susceptibility to chronic hepatitis B infection requires HLA genotyping-based association analysis. Scientific Reports. 2016;**6**:24767. DOI: 10.1038/srep24767

[29] Qiu B, Jiang W, Olyaee M, Shimura K, Miyakawa A, Hu H, et al. Advances in the genome-wide association study of chronic hepatitis B susceptibility in Asian population. European Journal of Medical Research. 2017;**22**(1):55. DOI: 10.1186/s40001-017-0288-3

[30] Liao X, Yu L, Liu X, Han C, Yu T, Qin W, et al. Genome-wide association pathway analysis to identify candidate singlenucleotide polymorphisms and molecular pathways associated with TP53 expression status in HBV-related hepatocellular carcinoma. Cancer Management and Research. 2018;**10**:953-967. DOI: 10.2147/CMAR.S163209

[31] Kang SS, Park WY, Jin K, Park SB, Han S. Characteristics of recipients with 10 or more years of allograft survival in deceased donor kidney transplantation. Transplantation Proceedings. 2018;**50**(4):1013-1017. DOI: 10.1016/j.transproceed.2018.02.040

[32] Kandilarova SM, Georgieva AI, Mihaylova AP, Baleva MP, Atanasova VK, Petrova DV, et al. Immune cell subsets evaluation as a predictive tool for hepatitis B infection outcome and treatment responsiveness. Folia Medica (Plovdiv). 2017;**59**(1):53-62. DOI: 10.1515/folmed-2017-0008

[33] van den Oord JJ, de Vos R, Desmet VJ. In situ distribution of major histocompatibility complex products and viral antigens in chronic hepatitis B virus infection: Evidence that HBc-containing hepatocytes may express HLA-DR antigens. Hepatology. 1986;**6**(5):981-989. PMID: 3530950

[34] Zhang SY, Gu HX, Li D, Yang SF, Zhong ZH, Li XK, et al. Association of HLA polymorphism with HBV infection and genotypes. Japanese Journal of Infectious Diseases. 2006;**59**(6):353-357. PMID: 17186951

[35] Tan W, Xia J, Dan Y, Li M, Lin S, Pan X, et al. Genome-wide association study identifies HLA-DR variants conferring risk of HBV-related acute-on-chronic liver failure. Gut. 2018;**67**(4):757-766. DOI: 10.1136/gutjnl-2016-313035

[36] Lin ZH, Xin YN, Dong QJ, Wang Q, Jiang XJ, Zhan SH, et al. Association between HLA-DRB1 alleles polymorphism and hepatocellular carcinoma: A meta-analysis. BMC Gastroenterology. 2010;**10**:145. DOI: 10.1186/1471-230X-10-145

[37] Ma S, Wu J, Wu J, Wei Y, Zhang L, Ning Q, et al. Relationship between HLA-DRB1 allele polymorphisms and familial aggregations of hepatocellular carcinoma. Current Oncology. 2016;**23**(1):e1-e7. DOI: 10.3747/co.23.2839

[38] Liu L, Guo W, Zhang J. Association of HLA-DRB1 gene polymorphisms with hepatocellular carcinoma risk: A meta-analysis. Minerva Medica. 2017;**108**(2):176-184. DOI: 10.23736/S0026-4806.16.04571-7

[39] Nishida N, Sawai H, Kashiwase K, Minami M, Sugiyama M, Seto WK, et al. New susceptibility and resistance HLA-DP alleles to HBV-related diseases identified by trans-ethnic association study in Asia. PLoS One. 2014;**9**(2):e86449. DOI: 10.1371/journal.pone.0086449

[40] Zhu M, Dai J, Wang C, Wang Y, Qin N, Ma H, et al. Fine mapping the MHC region identified four independent variants modifying susceptibility to chronic hepatitis B in Han Chinese. Human Molecular Genetics. 2016;**25**(6):1225-1232. DOI: 10.1093/hmg/ddw003

[41] Li S, Qian J, Yang Y, Zhao W, Dai J, Bei JX, et al. GWAS identifies novel susceptibility loci on 6p21.32 and 21q21.3 for hepatocellular carcinoma in chronic hepatitis B virus carriers. PLoS Genetics. 2012;**8**(7):e1002791. DOI: 10.1371/journal.pgen.1002791

[42] Wen J, Song C, Jiang D, Jin T, Dai J, Zhu L, et al. Hepatitis B virus genotype, mutations, human leukocyte antigen polymorphisms and their interactions in hepatocellular carcinoma: A multi-centre case-control study. Scientific Reports. 2015;5:16489. DOI: 10.1038/srep16489

[43] Jiang DK, Ma XP, Wu X, Peng L, Yin J, Dan Y, et al. Genetic variations in STAT4,C2,HLA-DRB1 and HLA-DQ associated with risk of hepatitis B virus-related liver cirrhosis. Scientific Reports. 2015;5:16278. DOI: 10.1038/srep16278

[44] Jiang DK, Sun J, Cao G, Liu Y, Lin D, Gao YZ, et al. Genetic variants in STAT4 and HLA-DQ genes confer risk of hepatitis B virus-related hepatocellular carcinoma. Nature Genetics. 2013;45(1):72-75. DOI: 10.1038/ng.2483

[45] Al-Qahtani AA, Al-Anazi MR, Abdo AA, Sanai FM, Al-Hamoudi W, Alswat KA, et al. Association between HLA variations and chronic hepatitis B virus infection in Saudi Arabian patients. PLoS One. 2014;9(1):e80445. DOI: 10.1371/journal.pone.0080445

[46] Zhang X, Jia J, Dong J, Yu F, Ma N, Li M, et al. HLA-DQ polymorphisms with HBV infection: Different outcomes upon infection and prognosis to lamivudine therapy. Journal of Viral Hepatitis. 2014;21(7):491-498. DOI: 10.1111/jvh.12159

[47] Xu T, Sun M, Wang H. Relationship between HLA-DQ gene polymorphism and hepatitis B virus infection. BioMed Research International. 2017;2017:9679843. DOI: 10.1155/2017/9679843

[48] Xu T, Zhu A, Sun M, Lv J, Qian Z, Wang X, et al. Quantitative assessment of HLA-DQ gene polymorphisms with the development of hepatitis B virus infection, clearance, liver cirrhosis, and hepatocellular carcinoma. Oncotarget. 2017;9(1):96-109. DOI: 10.18632/oncotarget.22941

[49] Chang SW, Fann CS, Su WH, Wang YC, Weng CC, Yu CJ, et al. A genome-wide association study on chronic HBV infection and its clinical progression in male Han-Taiwanese. PLoS One. 2014;9(6):e99724. DOI: 10.1371/journal.pone.0099724

[50] Kamatani Y, Wattanapokayakit S, Ochi H, Kawaguchi T, Takahashi A, Hosono N, et al. A genome-wide association study identifies variants in the HLA-DP locus associated with chronic hepatitis B in Asians. Nature Genetics. 2009;41(5):591-595. DOI: 10.1038/ng.348

[51] Howell JA, Visvanathan K. A novel role for human leukocyte antigen-DP in chronic hepatitis B infection: A genomewide association study. Hepatology. 2009;50(2):647-649. DOI: 10.1002/hep.23147

[52] Mohamadkhani A, Katoonizadeh A, Poustchi H. Immune-regulatory events in the clearance of HBsAg in chronic hepatitis B: Focuses on HLA-DP. Middle East Journal of Digestive Diseases. 2015;7(1):5-13. PMID: 25628847

[53] Wasityastuti W, Yano Y, Ratnasari N, Triyono T, Triwikatmani C, Indrarti F, et al. Protective effects of HLA-DPA1/DPB1 variants against hepatitis B virus infection in an Indonesian population. Infection, Genetics and Evolution. 2016;41:177-184. DOI: 10.1016/j.meegid.2016.03.034

[54] Akgöllü E, Bilgin R, Akkız H, Ülger Y, Kaya BY, Karaoğullarından Ü, et al. Association between chronic hepatitis B virus infection and HLA-DP gene polymorphisms in the Turkish population. Virus Research. 2017;**232**:6-12. DOI: 10.1016/j.virusres.2017.01.017

[55] Wang L, Wu XP, Zhang W, Zhu DH, Wang Y, Li YP, et al. Evaluation of genetic susceptibility loci for chronic hepatitis B in Chinese: Two independent case-control studies. PLoS One. 2011;**6**(3):e17608. DOI: 10.1371/journal.pone.0017608

[56] Nishida N, Sawai H, Matsuura K, Sugiyama M, Ahn SH, Park JY, et al. Genome-wide association study confirming association of HLA-DP with protection against chronic hepatitis B and viral clearance in Japanese and Korean. PLoS One. 2012;**7**(6):e39175. DOI: 10.1371/journal.pone.0039175

[57] O'Brien TR, Kohaar I, Pfeiffer RM, Maeder D, Yeager M, Schadt EE, et al. Risk alleles for chronic hepatitis B are associated with decreased mRNA expression of HLA-DPA1 and HLA-DPB1 in normal human liver. Genes and Immunity. 2011;**12**(6):428-433. DOI: 10.1038/gene.2011.11

[58] Vermehren J, Lötsch J, Susser S, Wicker S, Berger A, Zeuzem S, et al. A common HLA-DPA1 variant is associated with hepatitis B virus infection but fails to distinguish active from inactive Caucasian carriers. PLoS One. 2012;**7**(3):e32605. DOI: 10.1371/journal.pone.0032605

[59] Cheng HR, Liu CJ, Tseng TC, Su TH, Yang HI, Chen CJ, et al. Host genetic factors affecting spontaneous HBsAg seroclearance in chronic hepatitis B patients. PLoS One. 2013;**8**(1):e53008. DOI: 10.1371/journal.pone.0053008

[60] Liao Y, Cai B, Li Y, Chen J, Tao C, Huang H, et al. Association of HLA-DP/DQ and STAT4 polymorphisms with HBV infection outcomes and a minimeta-analysis. PLoS One. 2014;**9**(11):e111677. DOI: 10.1371/journal.pone.0111677

[61] Yu L, Cheng YJ, Cheng ML, Yao YM, Zhang Q, Zhao XK, et al. Quantitative assessment of common genetic variations in HLA-DP with hepatitis B virusinfection, clearance and hepatocellular carcinoma development. Scientific Reports. 2015;**5**:14933. DOI: 10.1038/srep14933

[62] Hu L, Zhai X, Liu J, Chu M, Pan S, Jiang J, et al. Genetic variants in human leukocyte antigen/DP-DQ influence both hepatitis B virus clearance and hepatocellular carcinoma development. Hepatology. 2012;**55**(5):1426-1431. DOI: 10.1002/hep.24799

[63] Thomas R, Thio CL, Apps R, Qi Y, Gao X, Marti D, et al. A novel variant marking HLA-DP expression levels predicts recovery from hepatitis B virusinfection. Journal of Virology. 2012;**86**(12):6979-6985. DOI: 10.1128/JVI.00406-12

[64] Hu Z, Yang J, Xiong G, Shi H, Yuan Y, Fan L, et al. HLA-DPB1 variant effect on hepatitis B virus clearance and liver cirrhosis development among southwest Chinese population. Hepatitis Monthly. 2014;**14**(8):e19747. DOI: 10.5812/hepatmon.19747

[65] The MHC sequencing consortium. Complete sequence and gene map of a human major histocompatibility complex. Nature. 1999;**401**(6756):921-923. PMID: 10553908

[66] Natarajan K, Jiang J, May NA, Mage MG, Boyd LF, McShan AC, et al. The role of molecular flexibility in antigen presentation and T cell receptor-mediated signaling. Frontiers in Immunology. 2018;**9**:1657. DOI: 10.3389/fimmu.2018.01657

[67] Wieczorek M, Abualrous ET, Sticht J, Álvaro-Benito M, Stolzenberg S, Noé F, et al. Major histocompatibility complex (MHC) class I and MHC class II proteins: Conformational plasticity in antigen presentation. Frontiers in Immunology. 2017;**8**:292. DOI: 10.3389/fimmu.2017.00292

[68] Misra MK, Damotte V, Hollenbach JA. Structure-based selection of human metabolite binding P4 pocket of DRB1*15:01 and DRB1*15:03, with implications for multiple sclerosis. Genes and Immunity. Jan 20, 2018. DOI: 10.1038/s41435-017-0009-5

[69] Hirasawa M, Hagihara K, Abe K, Ando O, Hirayama N. In silico and in vitro analysis of interaction between ximelagatran and human leukocyte antigen (HLA)-DRB1*07: 01. International Journal of Molecular Sciences. 2017;**18**(4):pii:E694. DOI: 10.3390/ijms18040694

[70] Hirasawa M, Hagihara K, Abe K, Ando O, Hirayama N. Interaction of nevirapine with the peptide binding groove of HLA-DRB1*01:01 and its effect on the conformation of HLA-peptide complex. International Journal of Molecular Sciences. 2018;**19**(6):pii: E1660. DOI: 10.3390/ijms19061660

[71] Delgado JC, Baena A, Thim S, Goldfeld AE. Aspartic acid homozygosity at codon 57 of HLA-DQ beta is associated with susceptibility to pulmonary tuberculosis in Cambodia. Journal of Immunology. 2006;**176**(2):1090-1097. DOI: https://doi.org/10.4049/jimmunol.176.2.1090

[72] Sun WX, Xia Y, Zhang SY. Crystal model of human Leukocyte antigen and its application in disease research. International Journal of Immunology. 2015;**38**(2):173-177. DOI: 10.3760/cma.j.issn.1673-4394.2015.02.017

[73] Xia Y, Sun WX, Li XK, Wang HY, Yu XY, Jin X, et al. Amino acids at positions 30β1 and 57β1 of HLA-DR confer susceptibility to or protection from chronic hepatitis B virus infection. International Journal of Clinical and Experimental Pathology. 2016;**9**(3):3816-3827. www.ijcep.com. ISSN: 1936-2625/IJCEP0020899

[74] Chow IT, James EA, Tan V, Moustakas AK, Papadopoulos GK, Kwok WW. DRB1*12:01 presents a unique subset of epitopes by preferring aromatics in pocket 9. Molecular Immunology. 2012;**50**(1-2):26-34. DOI: 10.1016/j.molimm.2011.11.014

[75] Stranger BE, Raj T. Genetics of human gene expression. Current Opinion in Genetics & Development. 2013;**23**(6):627-634. DOI: 10.1016/j.gde.2013.10.004

[76] Edwards JA, Durant BM, Jones DB, Evans PR, Smith JL. Differential expression of HLA class II antigens in fetal human spleen: Relationship of HLA-DP, DQ, and DR to immunoglobulin expression. Journal of Immunology. 1986;**137**(2):490-497. PMID: 3522732

[77] Pan W, Luo Q, Yan X, Yuan L, Yi H, Zhang L, et al. A novel SMAC mimetic APG-1387 exhibits dual antitumor effect on HBV-positive hepatocellular carcinoma with high expression of cIAP2 by inducing apoptosis and enhancing innate anti-tumor immunity. Biochemical Pharmacology. 2018;**154**:127-135. DOI: 10.1016/j.bcp.2018.04.020

[78] Jin X, Xia Y, Li XK, Wang D, Du B, Zhang SY. The characteristics of HLA-DR expression in patients with different outcomes of HBV infection. International Journal of Immunology. 2017;**40**(6):31-36. DOI: 10.3760/cma.j.issn.1673-4394.2017.06.007

[79] Dixon AL, Liang L, Moffatt MF, Chen W, Heath S, Wong KC, et al. A genome-wide association study of global gene expression. Nature Genetics. 2007;**39**(10):1202-1207. DOI: 10.1038/ng2109

[80] Emilsson V, Thorleifsson G, Zhang B, Leonardson AS, Zink F, Zhu J, et al. Genetics of gene expression and its effect on disease. Nature. 2008;**452**(7186):423-428. DOI: 10.1038/nature06758

[81] Schadt EE, Molony C, Chudin E, Hao K, Yang X, Lum PY, et al. Mapping the genetic architecture of gene expression in human liver. PLoS Biology. 2008;**6**(5):e107. DOI: 10.1371/journal.pbio.0060107

[82] Cavalli G, Hayashi M, Jin Y, Yorgov D, Santorico SA, Holcomb C, et al. MHC class II super-enhancer increases surface expression of HLA-DR and HLA-DQ and affects cytokine production in autoimmune vitiligo. Proceedings of the National Academy of Sciences of the United States of America. 2016;**113**(5):1363-1368. DOI: 10.1073/pnas.1523482113

[83] Kaur G, Gras S, Mobbs JI, Vivian JP, Cortes A, Barber T, et al. Structural and regulatory diversity shape HLA-C protein expression levels. Nature Communications. 2017;**8**:15924. DOI: 10.1038/ncomms15924

[84] Petersdorf EW, Malkki M, O'hUigin C, Carrington M, Gooley T, Haagenson MD, et al. High HLA-DP expression and graft-versus-host disease. The New England Journal of Medicine. 2015;**373**(7):599-609. DOI: 10.1056/NEJMoa1500140

[85] Schöne B, Bergmann S, Lang K, Wagner I, Schmidt AH, Petersdorf EW, et al. Predicting an HLA-DPB1 expression marker based on standard DPB1 genotyping: Linkage analysis of over 32,000 samples. Human Immunology. 2018;**79**(1):20-27. DOI: 10.1016/j.humimm.2017.11.001

[86] Wang X, Tang H, Teng M, Li Z, Li J, Fan J, et al. Mapping of hepatic expression quantitative trait loci (eQTLs) in a Han Chinese population. Journal of Medical Genetics. 2014;**51**(5):319-326. DOI: 10.1136/jmedgenet-2013-102045

[87] Nica AC, Dermitzakis ET. Expression quantitative trait loci: Present and future. Philosophical Transactions of the Royal Society of London. Series B, Biological Sciences. 2013;**368**(1620):20120362. DOI: 10.1098/rstb.2012.0362

[88] Zeng P, Zhou X, Huang S. Prediction of gene expression with cis-SNPs using mixed models and regularization methods. BMC Genomics. 2017;**18**(1):368. DOI: 10.1186/s12864-017-3759-6

[89] Zeng P, Wang T, Huang S. Cis-SNPs set testing and predixcan analysis for gene expression data using linear mixed models. Scientific Reports. 2017;**7**(1):15237. DOI: 10.1038/s41598-017-15055-8